BioSlim®

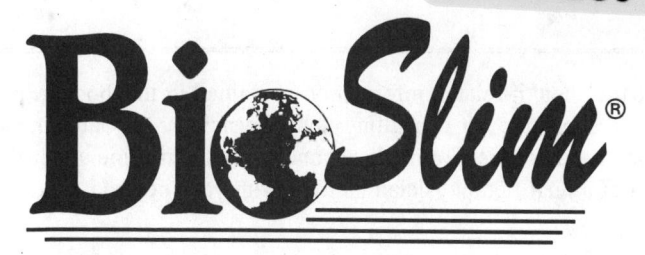

The *Natural* Total Health System

The Complete
DOCTOR'S REFERENCE GUIDE

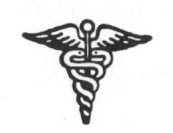

J. Leichtberg, M.D.

Any medical or health-related information contained in this book is not intended as a substitute for consulting your physician. Any attempt to diagnose or treat any illness or medical condition should come under the supervision of a qualified physician familiar with your personal medical history.

The information contained in this book, and the BioSlim program, are intended for use by normally healthy individuals as part of a general program of dietary and activity level improvement.

Designed and produced by J. Leichtberg, MD, BioSlim

BioSlim®, SlimTone Formula™, and Biotique™ are all trademarks of BioSlim

Copyright © 1993, 1994, 1997 J. Leichtberg, M.D., BioSlim

All rights reserved. No part of this publication may be reproduced, stored in a retrieval system, or transmitted, in any form or means, electronic, mechanical, photocopying, recording, or otherwise, without the prior written permission of the copyright owners.

Printed in the United States of America.

To my mother and father
whose never-ending efforts made it all possible;
to Forrest and Shanelle, the "babies", who make it all
worthwhile; and to their mother, for putting up with me

TABLE OF CONTENTS

SECTION ONE
WHY BIOSLIM?

1. **INTRODUCTION** 2
   - You've Got Lots of Company! 4
   - Solution: Linking Weight Loss to Health 4
2. **WHY IS THERE FAT AND WHAT IS IT?** 6
   - Why Is There Fat 6
   - Obesity Defined 7
   - Finding Out Where You Stand 8
   - BMI: A Useful Measure of Weight Status 9
   - Where Your Fat Lies Matters! 9
   - What Happens When You Diet 10
   - Scale vs. Mirror 10
   - Keeping It Simple and Fun 11
3. **WHY DO WE BECOME OVERWEIGHT?** 12
   - Fat Cells, Dieting and Metabolism 12
   - Carbohydrates and Carbohydrate Intolerance 13
   - Fat and How It Affects Your Body 14
   - Controlling Your Body's Fat 16
4. **THE CONSEQUENCES OF BEING OVERWEIGHT** 18
5. **YOUR CHOICES: WEIGHT CONTROL REVIEW** 20
   - The Options You've Had *(before BioSlim)* 20
   - The Government and the Diet Industry 20
   - If Not BioSlim, What? 22
   - Powders, Shakes, "Diet" Bars and Other Nonsense 22

i

"Meal Replacements": Tickets to Failure............. 23
"Designer" Diets: Atkins, et al................................ 24
Drugs.. 26
Surgery... 27
Only Right Way to Healthful, Permanent Weight
Control 28

6. WHAT IS BIOSLIM? **29**
Dieting Fact Review 30
Your Goals with BioSlim... 32

7. THE BEGINNING: WHY CHANGE IS ESSENTIAL **35**
BioSlim and the Medical Group.................................... 35
Suffer the Children... 36
What Happens as the Child Grows: The Frequent
Inevitability of Obesity.. 38
What Is Right and What Is Wrong with the Way
We Eat—What to Do About It...................................... 40

8. WHEN THE SCALE ALWAYS RISES: REACTIONS............ **44**
"Who Cares?" 44
The Self-Destructive Impulse.. 45
The "Hopelessly Hungry" Syndrome 47
"Oh well, I tried...".. 47
Review of Weight Reaction Categories........................ 48
Solutions 49

9. THE BEST, MOST HEALTHFUL WAY TO ACHIEVE
YOUR OPTIMAL WEIGHT... **50**
Staying Happy: Vital to Success................................... 51

SECTION TWO
THE BIOSLIM PRINCIPLES

---

10. MEDICAL CONSIDERATIONS **53**
Ten Things to Say to Your Doctor to Help
Improve Your Health 54

Ten Warning Signs to Watch For in Your
Doctor..55
♦ Adrenal gland dysfunction...............................56
♦ Aging..57
♦ Allergies and substance sensitivities................58
♦ Anemia...59
♦ Arthritis..60
♦ Asthma...62
♦ Back pain...62
♦ Cancer..63
♦ Carpal tunnel syndrome...................................65
♦ Cataracts..65
♦ Cholesterol level, elevated...............................66
♦ Colitis...69
♦ Constipation...72
♦ Diabetes...73
♦ Fatigue, chronic or severe................................75
♦ Gallstones..78
♦ Hay fever...78
♦ Headaches..79
♦ Heart disease / Cardiovascular disorders.........81
♦ Hemorrhoids..83
♦ High Blood Pressure (hypertension)................84
♦ Kidney Stones..85
♦ Lung disorders...86
♦ Multiple Sclerosis (MS)...................................88
♦ Osteoporosis..89
♦ Pregnancy..90
♦ Prostate enlargement..91
♦ Skin wrinkling...92
♦ Stress..92
♦ Thyroid gland disease......................................93
♦ Ulcers (stomach and duodenal)........................96
♦ Vaginitis / Yeast infections..............................98

11. NEVER "GO ON A DIET" AGAIN!..............................100

12. THE BIOSLIM FOOD PLAN: EAT ALL THE REAL, GOOD FOOD YOU WANT ... 102
   Essential Principles of BioSlim Food Plan ... 103
   Food Rating Guide ... 110
      The Right Stuff - I ... 111
      The Right Stuff - II ... 113
      Foods To Avoid ... 116
   Salt ... 119
   About Water ... 119
   Coffee ... 120
   Food Preparation ... 120
   Spirulina for Breakfast? ... 121
   When to Eat; When to Stop ... 122
   Restaurant Eating ... 122
   Cheating ("indulging") ... 124

13. NUTRITION: THE KEY TO HEALTH ... 126
   Nutrition ... 126
   Digestion ... 127
   Metabolism ... 128
   Food Components: Where Calories Come From ... 129
      Proteins ... 130
      Carbohydrates ... 131
      Fats ... 132
   VITAMINS ... 135
      Vitamin A ... 136
      The B Vitamins ... 137
      Vitamin C (Ascorbic Acid) ... 138
      Vitamin D ... 139
      Vitamin E ... 140
      Vitamin K ... 140
      Bioflavonoids ... 140
   Minerals ... 141
   Other Nutrients ... 143
   Dangerous Products ... 143

14. THE BIOSLIM FORMULAS ... 145
   SlimTone Formula ... 146

Vita/Min Plus 147
What effect? 148
Optional: Adding Nutrients 150

15. THE ACTIVITY PLAN **152**
Diet and Activity 154
Basic Activity Plan Tips 155

16. THE SECRET POWER INSIDE YOU **157**

17. MASTERING MOTIVATION **162**
We Are All OK 164
A Way To Eat 165
Separating Real Hunger From False Hunger 166
Taking Action 169
Thirst is Not Hunger 174
Naturally Thin 175
Mental Tools 175
Course Corrections 177
The Vicious Circle and How to End It 179

18. WHAT TO DO ABOUT THOSE CRAVINGS **180**
Why We Get Cravings, Physically 181
How to Prevent and Stop Cravings 185

19. MAINTAINING YOUR ACHIEVEMENTS **189**
How It's Done 189

20. SOLVING PROBLEMS **191**
I. Weight Loss is Too Slow 191
Ia. When to Use *Super BioSlim* 194
II. Weight Loss is Too Rapid 195
III. Energy Level is Not High Enough 195
IV. Energy Level is Too High 196
V. Your Digestive Tract 197
   • Constipation or Diarrhea 197
   • Intestinal Gas 197
VI. When to See Your Doctor 198

21. WOMEN: SPECIAL FACTS AND CONSIDERATIONS .. **199**
The Thyroid: Nothing Works if it Does Not 199

Special Nutritional Requirements 199
The Body 200
Iron / Anemia 201
Pregnancy 201
Menstrual Changes 202
Menopause 202
Yeast Syndromes 203

22. THE FUTURE 205

SECTION THREE
APPENDIX

FOODS AT A GLANCE 207
General Guidelines Review 207
Samples: Quick Snacks 208
Samples: Good Breakfast Choices 209
Samples: Lunch and Dinner 209
Vegetables 210
Fruit 211
High Protein Foods 211
High-Carbohydrate Foods 211
Fast Food Outlets 212
Tips 212

THE SUPER BIOSLIM PLAN 213
How *Super BioSlim* Works 214

INDEX 217

SECTION ONE

WHY BIOSLIM?

One

INTRODUCTION

This book is about three very important aspects of your life: how much fat your body carries, how you eat and the state of your health.

While it may seem intuitively obvious that these issues are closely interrelated, the fact is that our society mostly ignores these vital relationships. People too often go to doctors with their ills only to receive high-tech, often potentially dangerous, usually expensive tests and drugs for their trouble. We rarely hear about diet and lifestyle from the medical community.

But others *do* find these issues important and interesting; reports on the links between diet and various aspects of health and well-being appear often in the press and electronic media. And various self-proclaimed "experts" have taken up the task of teaching the public about health, diet and nutrition. The moral and educational duty often abandoned by the medical profession has been assumed in part by an array of untrained, ill-informed business-people who—prior to finding their pot of gold in the health and diet business—may have worked in comedy, or as actors, or in some cases, were simply overweight folks who managed to lose some weight and found a knack for salesmanship.

And so it goes: doctors continue to prescribe ever more expensive and powerful drugs and procedures, while the public is "taught" basic nutrition by the news media, or by business-people far more concerned with their bankbooks than with imparting accurate, useful information.

Unfortunately, lessons learned from the six-o'clock news are quickly forgotten. And information gathered from the other dubious sources on the market today is mostly unreliable, even potentially dangerous.

What we get as a result of all this are intermittent mass cholesterol-phobias, cancer scares, people who are afraid to eat *anything* and a public whose knowledge of nutrition and preventive medicine is rudimentary and too general, lacking as it does the kind of personalization that can and should come from the one-on-one attention of trained health care practitioners.

So where are people supposed to get the information they need to normalize weight, live healthfully and avoid the chronic diseases that plague our society? Not usually from their drug-oriented, nutritionally uninformed doctors; they are neither trained nor do they, for the most part, care very much about diet and nutrition. Not in any meaningful way from the news media. Certainly not from the hucksters and manipulators in the diet industry. And not in our schools, where "nutrition" is still often defined as the "four basic food groups" (a now discredited notion promulgated originally by the meat and dairy industries to sell more of their products).

One way is by reading about nutrition and health in books—like this one.

It is time now for at least some of us in the medical profession to reassume our rightful and vital responsibility to inform the public how to best care for its health and how to *prevent* illness. That is what we must focus on—not, as is too often the case today, on a never-ending stream of esoteric, marginally effective new technology and drugs.

So it is the purpose of this book to provide the reader with the knowledge and tools necessary to the achievement of optimal weight, health and well-being. While the central focus is on achieving a proper and healthful weight, the overriding issue remains *health,* for health and life are but two sides of the same coin.

4 ♦ *Why BioSlim?*

YOU'VE GOT LOTS OF COMPANY!

Polls show that between 52% and 70% of all Americans believe they need to lose weight. Over 50% of all Americans are overweight. This is a HUGE problem—the single most prevalent health risk in America today. And it gets worse every year. At this rate, it is estimated that by the year 2230 virtually *everyone* will be too fat!

Dieting has become a national obsession. Two out of every three adults consume some form of diet food each year. Americans spend an estimated **$40 *billion*** on diets and diet aids each year—an amazing sum. And what does all this achieve?

Very little.

Almost nothing.

The unhappy truth is that virtually *everyone* who "goes on a diet" to lose weight will either fail to achieve his or her goals, or, if the weight goal is somehow achieved, will eventually regain all the lost weight. In many cases, the "bounce-back" effect will cause a weight gain *greater* than the original weight loss. This process, commonly known as "yo-yo" dieting, has been found in several studies to be *itself* dangerous to human health—a danger that is *in addition* to the risks inherent in the overweight state.

The fact is: **losing weight is not the difficult issue in obesity**. There are many ways of doing it, as we will see below. ***Keeping the weight off*** is where the true difficulty lies. Fully 95% to 99% of all dieters regain their lost weight—a truly astounding statistic! Astounding and sad in the scope of futility it reflects.

SOLUTION: LINKING WEIGHT LOSS TO HEALTH

We must view the goal of weight loss as part of a larger picture, as integrated into the process of achieving good health, not as an isolated problem in need of a solution. It is this latter, narrower view of weight control that is the fundamental problem with most of today's weight loss methods. Like so many aspects of health care in America today, weight control has too often been approached as an *acute care* kind of problem—i.e., "fix it when it happens"—instead of addressing the issue with concern for the *whole* body and taking steps to not only cure but *prevent* the problem in the first place.

If normalization of weight is achieved through the *health-building* methods outlined in this book, overall health can benefit enormously along with the weight control achieved. To this end, this book does not offer quick-fix, impermanent ways to achieve weight loss. That kind of approach—the one you are unfortunately probably most familiar with—simply cannot in good faith be recommended.

There are no strange "magic" diets schemes here. No esoteric foods, shakes or powders to buy or eat. No dangerous starvation "diets". No unnecessary deprivation. Instead, BioSlim is about *losing* weight by *gaining* good health. It's about allowing your body to normalize itself by giving it the nutrients and support it needs.

As your body becomes healthier it will find its balance. It is in that balance that you will achieve each and every one of your health and body goals, and most importantly, *maintain* them.

Now let's get to the how's and wherefores.

> AUTHOR'S NOTE: The *Super BioSlim Plan,* in the *Appendix,* is a new addition. It is a powerful plan to help the most difficult of cases achieve their goals, and will result in rapid weight loss. It is a more temporary measure, meant to be used when the user requires even more power than the standard BioSlim plan provides to begin his or her program. A gradual transition to the regular BioSlim plan is always recommended.

Two

WHY IS THERE FAT and WHAT IS IT?

WHY IS THERE FAT

Believe it or not, fat is important. It is not nature's mistake, but rather, *essential to life.* The ability to store energy in the form of fat is a critical survival mechanism for any living organism subject to an uncertain and intermittently inadequate food supply. Humans can survive up to two months with no food whatsoever—in total starvation, with only water—only because of the presence of stored energy in the body, mostly in the form of fat. Fat is by far the body's most efficient method for storing energy. And body fat also provides shielding from cold.

Body fat is stored in response to insulin. Insulin is released from the pancreas in response to high blood sugar levels. You get high blood sugar after eating sugar (though much less so with fructose), or high-carbohydrate foods like all flour products (pasta, bread, cake, etc.) You can see, then, why it is so important to avoid *unbalanced* food plans—where insulin levels are too high and body fat is stored too readily, burned too rarely.

In particular, high lab levels of *serum triglycerides* often indicate too much insulin in the system too often, a condition known as *hyperinsulinemia* ("high blood insulin"). If this is your situation, you MUST follow the BioSlim Food Plan as closely as possible, matching carbohydrate intake to protein intake, and avoiding all sugars and concentrated carbohydrate foods such as flour and grain products, potatoes, corn, undiluted fruit juices, etc.—as described in the *BioSlim Food Plan* chapter below. There is much more information on this subject in *Chapter 3* below (*Why Do We Become Overweight?*).

Certain dietary fats are essential for proper body function. These are known, appropriately enough, as the *Essential Fatty Acids* (more on these "EFAs" later). And there is some form of fat (as well as *cholesterol*) in every single cell of your body.

Unfortunately, in most of Western society, many of the survival advantages nature intended fat to provide are unneeded. Food is typically not scarce, but abundant and in constant supply. Most people do not require an "energy reservoir", as they too often lead quite sedentary lives.

As a result, the body's ability to store fat has become more a problem than a survival mechanism. The problem is *obesity*.

OBESITY DEFINED

"Obesity" remains an imprecisely defined word. It is best viewed as any degree of excess body fat storage that imparts a health risk. By that definition, using the best data available, a person can be termed obese if he or she is approximately 20% above ideal weight. Of course, "ideal" weight is also imprecisely defined, but can be estimated from body type and actuarial tables, or, perhaps best of all, by using a mirror (see below).

You can define your own situation very easily if you know how much weight you need to lose to get to what you consider your ideal state. Take that number, divide it by your ideal weight, and the resultant fraction is the percentage by which you are above your ideal weight. If it's more than 20%—or even 10%!—read on: you need to do something about it.

This brings up an important and very useful alternative definition of obesity—the overweight state—provided by that highly informative article of home furnishing, the *mirror*. Most of us can take one look in a mirror, and by comparing what we see with what we remember from when we were either younger or healthier or both, we know quite well whether or not we need to lose weight, and a fair idea of how much.

Some people may fit the "optimal height/weight" charts perfectly, but are nevertheless clearly overweight by the "mirror criteria". Others may be obese according to the charts but are clearly not so by the mirror test (usually due to increased muscularity or frame size).

Note that muscle is much *denser* (heavier per unit volume) than fat, so that a muscular body may easily weigh far more than the charts recommend, yet be perfectly appropriate and healthy.

FINDING OUT WHERE YOU STAND

One effective way to determine your status is to undergo a *body fat analysis*. While there are several ways to accomplish this, including very elaborate and expensive methods, there are now two simple, inexpensive ways, one of which can be recommended. The first is *anthropometry*, which includes the use of calipers to measure skin fold thickness, typically in the upper arm and back areas. This method is extremely simple, but the results are highly variable and generally unreliable, particularly if done on oneself or by non-professionals. You can get *some* general idea of your status with this, but don't rely on it.

The other, much-preferred method is called *electrolipography*. It involves a 3 to 4 minute procedure whereby electrodes are attached to the hands and feet and a measurement taken—much the way an EKG (electrocardiogram) is performed. It is painless and perfectly safe. It relies on the observation that higher body fat content presents a greater resistance to electrical flow. By integrating statistical data about height, weight, age, sex and the electrolipograph test results, a surprisingly accurate measure of body fat can be obtained. Results from this test are quite reproducible, and if care is taken to obtain accurate measurements, it can be an excellent way to not only perform a one-time body fat analysis, but to follow the progress of an individual's percentage of body fat.

Your "percentage of body fat" is defined simply as the percentage of your body that is fat. "Percentage of lean body weight" means the percentage of your body that is "lean", or made up mostly of muscle tissue. Testing for body fat is more desirable for following your progress on any weight control system than simply charting your weight, since it is *fat* that most people need to lose, not merely weight. As we shall see, it is very easy to lose *muscle* through dieting, instead of fat—a highly undesirable, self-defeating outcome that is all too common under most of today's commercially available diet plans (see *What Happens When You Diet* below).

Body fat analysis is generally available at health clubs and some health practitioners' (doctors, chiropractors, etc.) offices.

Keep in mind: This is a useful tool, but *not at all* essential to the BioSlim program. The decision on whether to use it or not is a matter of personal choice and need. You can do just fine without it.

BMI: A USEFUL MEASURE OF WEIGHT STATUS

BMI (Body Mass Index) is a useful measure of your weight status as it relates to health risks. It is calculated by taking your weight *in kilograms* (1 kilogram = 2.2 pounds), and dividing it by the *square* of your height *in meters* (1 meter = 39.37 inches, or 3.28 feet).

For example, if you weigh 170 pounds, that's 170÷2.2= 77.3 kilograms. If you're 6 foot tall (72 inches), that would be 72÷39.37= 1.83 meters. Multiply 1.83x1.83 (the *square* of your height in meters) to get 3.34. Divide 77.3 by 3.34 = 23.14.

Any BMI under 25 is considered OK. Over 27 is generally considered obese. In between is a gray area—you could be overweight, or stockily built.

BMI is a useful measure, but not the gold standard. That remains your actual percentage of body fat. And: no test is better than the simple mirror test we all know so well.

WHERE YOUR FAT LIES MATTERS!

When excess body fat is stored above the waist (e.g., "pot belly"), as is commonly the case in overweight men, the danger to health is greater than when the fat is stored below the waist (hips, thighs), as is the case for most overweight women. It is believed that this is due to the type of fat stored in these areas: the above-the-waist fat seems to be more unstable, more hyperactive, and appears to break off more easily to attach itself in other areas via the bloodstream.

WHAT HAPPENS WHEN YOU DIET

Severely restrictive diets, such as "liquid protein" diets, or some of the popular "crash" diet programs—or any diet that recommends shakes or powders or drinks or candy bars instead of meals—can cause unhealthful weight loss that is too often due in large part to *lean body weight loss*, or loss of important body muscle mass, as well as an initially rapid, potentially dangerous loss of body water. This kind of weight loss is the worst possible way to achieve your goals because it is a) impermanent, and b) leads to weakness, ill health, and a *decreased metabolic rate* resulting from having fewer "furnaces" in which to burn calories (muscles are where energy is used up, or "burned").

This decreased metabolic rate makes it harder to lose weight. This, then, sets up the never-ending cycle of defeat and futility so familiar to the chronic dieter. (See Chapter 5, *Your Choices: Weight Control Review,* for more on this important issue.)

SCALE VS. MIRROR

As you progress in your BioSlim program, particularly if you fully and enthusiastically incorporate the Activity Plan, you may find that your clothes are getting looser and you're feeling terrific — yet your weight drops by only a small amount on some weeks. That may well be because your *lean body mass*, i.e., muscle mass, is growing at a rate that is faster than the one at which your body fat is diminishing; i.e., you're getting stronger! Conversely, if you restrict your eating too severely, as on many "diet" programs, you may lose weight during some weeks, but your *percentage of body fat* may not improve, and may even rise, despite your weight loss.

Note: Body fat analysis, as we have seen, is a good way to accurately track your progress, but is not easy to find. Therefore, *don't worry if you can't have it done.* Most people can't. Use your mirror! By combining the information it gives with how your clothes fit, you will have quite an accurate and sensitive guide to how you're doing on the program. Yes, your scale is useful. But remember: it has its limitations, the most significant of which is its inability to differentiate between *good* weight loss (*fat* loss) and *bad* weight loss (loss of *lean* body mass).

KEEPING IT SIMPLE AND FUN

There is another fundamentally good reason for why, if it is not readily available, we recommend you *not* search for a way to have body fat analysis done. It is a central principle of BioSlim that nothing about the program be difficult or unpleasant in any way. If you create a system for yourself that is something you feel you have to "suffer through for a while"—a temporary unpleasantness you will stoically bear in order to lose some weight—then, *by definition,* you intend to someday stop the program and go back to your old ways. When you do that, there is only one thing that can happen: you will regain the weight you lost (and perhaps a little more, as we shall see).

So KEEP THIS PROGRAM SIMPLE AND FUN. Do this for yourself—because it is the only way to know for sure that you'll stick to the program.

Please remember as you read this book: the purpose of BioSlim is to help you achieve *permanent, healthful weight loss.* You should strive to remove from your life anything that may get in the way of that goal, including anything that is, within reason, burdensome to you.

THREE

WHY DO WE BECOME OVERWEIGHT?
ଔଓ

Why *do* people become overweight? This is a question without a completely satisfactory answer, as some of the pieces of the puzzle continue to elude medical science. What we know:

FAT CELLS, DIETING AND METABOLISM

- It is believed that the number of fat cells ("adipocytes") in the body never diminishes. You can *gain* fat cells, particularly in childhood. But once gained, they don't seem to ever go away or diminish *in number*. For years, it had been thought that the number of fat cells in the body is set in childhood, and that adults cannot alter that number, only the size of the fat cells (which can shrink to almost nothing).

- When adults become obese, their existing fat cells dramatically increase *in size* to hold the extra fat. And it now appears, contrary to the previously held notions described above, that adults may also gain new fat cells as they grow obese. In any event, once gained, fat cells never disappear, though they do change in size.

- *Dieting,* or the restriction of calorie intake, causes a *reduction* of metabolic rate. (*Metabolic rate* is the speed at which the body's engine runs and at which it burns calories.) This is the body's way of conserving energy in the face of what it perceives to be a period of starvation. Remember, your body was designed to withstand the intermittent food shortages of primeval times by storing fat. When you diet, your body doesn't know you're trying to lose weight. It reacts by slowing down body functions, and *speeding up fat storage*, so as to both conserve energy and store it (in the form of fat) for future use. In this very real sense, **DIETING MAKES YOU FATTER!!** — not thinner.

- *"Basal"* metabolism, the body's metabolism at rest, accounts for approximately 70% of all energy expenditures in a normal individual. It represents the energy your body uses just to stay alive: breathing, heart beating, brain working, heat production, etc. Exercise may raise the *non-resting* use of energy, but as you can see, its effect cannot be greater than that of the underlying basal metabolism necessary to vital body function. However, there is evidence now that regular activity increases not only the rate of calorie use *during* activity, but also the *resting* metabolic rate *afterwards*, which dramatically alters the equation.

- The basal (resting) metabolism of an otherwise normally healthy obese individual is not typically different from that of a healthy non-obese person. Of course, there are significant medical conditions that can lead to an overweight state, as discussed in the *Medical Considerations* chapter below.

- Some medications will make you gain weight. Examples: tricyclic antidepressants, antihistamines (especially astemizole and loratadine), and corticosteroids (aka, "steroids").

Carbohydrates and Carbohydrate Intolerance

- Approximately 25% of the population are intolerant to high levels of carbohydrates in the diet. If you are in this group and you eat a typical Western diet of high carbohydrates (flour products, sugars, starches) and high added fat, you are virtually certain to become obese. One clue to this condition is your blood level of *triglycerides*, a kind of blood fat. If high, it tends to indicate a state of *hyperinsulinemia*, or high insulin levels. Insulin is the hormone that tells your body to store fat and burn less fat for energy. Insulin also reduces blood levels of *growth hormone*—a pituitary hormone that, among other things, causes more fat to be burned for energy, creating a leaner healthier body, and is believed to help forestall the effects of aging.

- Sugar is one of the worst offenders when it comes to increasing body fat (and insulin levels). Note that *fructose*, a kind of sugar, is much more slowly absorbed into the bloodstream than sucrose (table sugar), and is therefore far less likely to undesirably affect insulin levels and body fat storage.
- Too much alcohol can slow down fat metabolism and make you fatter. Suggestion: up to one glass of wine per day is OK.
- Foods that contain high levels of rapidly-absorbed carbohydrates tend to do the most damage when it comes to elevating insulin levels and making you fatter. They should be avoided, especially if you are carbohydrate intolerant. These include:
  * Grains, including rice, corn and all flour products such as bread, pasta, cake, etc. If you must eat grains, eat only *whole* grains, such as oatmeal, whole wheat, brown rice, etc.
  * A few vegetables, such as potatoes, carrot, beet
  * Sweet fruits, especially banana, papaya, undiluted fruit juices, raisins, grapes
  * High-sugar foods, e.g. candies, other sweets, soft drinks, etc.

FAT AND HOW IT AFFECTS YOUR BODY

- Eating fat, especially *added* fat (fat that is added to food, as opposed to the fat that is naturally present in real food), does all kinds of damage to your body, including increasing your risk of heart disease, cancer, diabetes, high blood pressure, and many other unpleasant things. It also makes you fatter faster than anything else you can eat, containing as it does over twice the calories (9 per gram) by weight as the other food constituents (4 per gram for protein or carbohydrate).

  Excess fat ingestion also appears to increase "insulin resistance", a condition where more and more insulin must be supplied to the body as the tissues become more and more immune to its effects. This can greatly exacerbate the problem of obesity, and can lead to diabetes.

- Fat is not all bad. Here's why (see also Chapter 2, *Why Is There Fat...*):

  Fat makes you feel fuller faster. This is partly due to its slow digestion, as well as to its causing the release of *cholecystokinin* ("CCK") a stomach hormone that tells your brain: you're full, stop eating. Fat that appears naturally in food need not be avoided; it actually helps control appetite.

  Fat slows digestion of virtually *all* food eaten with it... especially carbohydrates. Fat that appears naturally in food will help slow down carbohydrate absorption, thereby reducing what might otherwise be a flood of insulin responding to a flood of carbohydrates entering the bloodstream.

  Monounsaturated fats are the best fats to eat. Found in high levels in olives and olive oil, avocados, macadamia nuts and canola oil, these fats have actually been linked to *reduced* heart disease and cancer rates. However...

  Note: Olive oil and canola oils are still oils! They are still pure fat. And they are still added fats, meaning nature does not create olive or canola oil. The body will *not* react well to having these unnaturally produced, *added* fats thrown into it, no matter the potential beneficial effects on one disease or another. However, if you *must* use an added fat or oil, these two oils are the best to use, especially olive oil. But remember: *all added fats should be avoided* for maximum benefit under the BioSlim plan.

- The response of an obese person's metabolism to food is quite different from that of a non-obese individual: it is usually not as robust—not as aggressive. Food, *particularly food high in oil and fat,* will make an obese person gain weight *faster* than it will a thin person. This is in part due to the observed reduction in obese individuals of *food-induced thermogenesis,* which is the body's increase in heat production in response to food ingestion ("thermogenesis" means "heat production"). It is one of the reasons you may feel warmer after a meal. Subjects who are overweight have been observed to have a generally <u>weaker</u> food-induced thermogenesis response than lean individuals. This is a form of reduced metabolic rate, though it is only part of the whole picture.

Note that the food-induced thermogenesis effect is most significant when the ingested food is a carbohydrate or a protein, and *least* noticeable when it is fat. So not only is fat higher in calories gram for gram than carbohydrates or protein, it apparently also *reduces the body's ability to burn up calories* through food-induced heat production. In fact, as we have seen, ingested fat tends to induce the body to *store* calories—as body fat. This is one more important reason to avoid added fats in the diet. ***Fat makes you fat.***

Controlling Your Body's Fat

- Childhood habits and adult eating patterns appear to have the most direct influence on adult body fat levels. If you learned in childhood to "always clean your plate", you will probably carry that programming with you into adulthood. If you were heavy as a child, your chances of being an overweight adult are much higher than they would otherwise be. It is possible to break the physical and psychological programming of childhood—but it is not a simple matter. The BioSlim program is the single best way to do this, as it was designed with this very purpose in mind.

- There appears to be an appetite control center in the brain that governs the overeating that accompanies many cases of obesity. There is no known *direct* way to alter its function.

- Emotional states such as anger, depression, fear of success and reactions to stress all can and do contribute to the onset and promotion of the overweight state A condition known as SAD (*Seasonal Affective Disorder*), affecting approximately 10 million Americans, causes depression and often weight gain in fall and winter—when our daily dose of sunlight diminishes. Going outdoors more, avoiding sunglasses, and treatment with light (done professionally) all can help alleviate the symptoms of SAD.

- Anaerobic exercise (such as isometrics or weight lifting) tends to increase growth hormone levels, with all the salutary effect that can have, including the faster and more efficient use of body fat for energy, the strengthening of body muscles, and, apparently, improvements in many of the effects of aging.

- New research indicates there may be a "fat gene" that makes some of us obese. If so, people with this gene simply must be more careful and attentive to their health than others. The vast majority of overweight Americans appear to *not* have this genetic predisposition. Their weight problems can be traced to their food, activity and nutritional practices.

* * *

There is no one simple answer to the question of why people become overweight. For some, it is due to physical or medical factors, such as hormonal or metabolic disorders, or medications. For others, it is because of psychological issues like self-image and interpersonal relationships. There are as many answers as there are people with the problem. And each, like most things concerning the human experience, is a complex mix of physical, emotional, and environmental factors.

In this book, we will focus on ways to bring balance and *sense* to this difficult, troubling issue.

We will *not* try to force you into a preconceived mold. You will find within the BioSlim system answers that are right—*perfect*—for you. The key words here are: *"you will find...".* With a problem this complex and this personal, the only good answers are the ones *you* discover are right *for you*.

We will give you the facts and recommend healthful, permanent solutions. But *you* must decide to implement them, and you must feel right about using them.

So keep reading: the right answers will soon be clear and obvious to you. It should feel *right*, and should make you *happy*.

DO IT!... for yourself.

THE CONSEQUENCES OF BEING OVERWEIGHT

ೞ೮

Below is a list of the most common serious problems for which carrying too much body weight increases your risk.

Details on the medical aspects of body weight and its relationship to various specific health issues are presented in the *Medical Considerations* chapter.

The following list conveys the general scope of the problem.

- High blood pressure
- Diabetes
- Heart disease
- Lung disease
- Breathing disorders
- Cancer, such as of the breast, colon and uterus
- Atherosclerosis (hardening of the arteries)
- High cholesterol and triglyceride levels
- Liver disease (fatty liver)
- Osteoarthritis (especially of the hips)
- Sciatica or other spinal pain syndromes
- Gout
- Gallstones
- Gallbladder inflammation
- Blood clots
- Toxemia of pregnancy
- Menstrual irregularities
- Various hernias

- Sleep disorders
- Growth hormone suppression
- ...and sudden death

Each of these can be ameliorated by proper weight control. Some, particularly the cardiovascular effects and diabetes, are actually exacerbated by repeated "yo-yo" dieting, i.e., they can get *worse* if your weight constantly fluctuates up and down.

With all this, one may conclude that weight loss is perhaps not the most important reason to get on—and stay on—the BioSlim program. Looking at the list above, would not the more important reason be your health and how long you're going to live?

This is, in fact, the best way to think about BioSlim: do it for your health—for *life*. If you follow the BioSlim system with these thoughts in mind, the excess weight will **melt from your body.** Don't worry about the weight... it WILL come off! Concentrate on *doing the right thing.* Your body will take care of itself— it has an amazing ability to do just that. All you have to do is give it a chance.

* * *

Now, before we begin exploring the BioSlim system, let us review the available *alternatives.*

FIVE

YOUR CHOICES: WEIGHT CONTROL REVIEW
☙❧

"Destiny is not a matter of chance, it is a matter of choice."

THE OPTIONS YOU'VE HAD *(before BioSlim)*

It is important now to review the other ways available to you for weight loss. By understanding the facts about each of these methods—why each one fails in its own way—you will also clearly see why the approach embodied in the BioSlim system is the one that must be right for you.

We will review these general categories of weight loss methods:
- Powders, Shakes, "Diet" Bars (e.g., "Pounds Off" bars) and other nonsense
- "Meal Replacements"
- "Designer" Diets, including Atkins, #-Day Diets, etc.
- Drugs
- Surgery
- Liposuction, tucks, and other such options

We will then see how BioSlim overcomes the problems these methods create and how BioSlim brings to you the ultimate, *permanent* answer to the "diet dilemma".

THE GOVERNMENT AND THE DIET INDUSTRY

In 1990 congressional hearings were held that focused attention on the weight-loss claims made by various diet companies. In October, 1991, the FTC (Federal Trade

Commission) fired its first shot against the industry when it took action against three liquid diet makers: Optifast, Medifast and Ultrafast. These three companies agreed at that time to drop certain claims they had been making about the safety and effectiveness of their products.

It was explained then by the FTC that these severely calorie-restricted diets (a) were potentially dangerous, and (b) virtually *never* work permanently. The companies involved were forced to drop the claims they had been making about "fast, easy, long-term weight loss" because they were determined to be false by the U.S. government.

In 1993, the FTC disclosed it is investigating several more companies, including the biggest ones in the industry, for their false and misleading advertising. As before, the FTC believed their claims of "fast, easy, long-lasting" weight loss were in fact false and misleading.

The companies investigated by the FTC include:
- Jenny Craig, Inc.,
- Nutri/System Inc.,
- Weight Watchers International,
- Diet Centers, and
- Physicians Weight Loss Centers.

Other investigated companies/programs include: Health Management Resources' *Fasting Program*; United Weight Control Corporation's *Permanence Program* and *Risk Reduction Program*; and Abbott Laboratories' *New Directions*.

According to the FTC, all appear to practice false and misleading advertising when they claim that their programs are safe, effective, and most significantly and most falsely, *permanent,* which, of course, virtually *none* are.

Let's now review some of the various commercially available weight control programs. We will see that what is wrong with most of them is approximately what the FTC found wrong with the companies mentioned above.

IF NOT BIOSLIM, WHAT?

POWDERS, SHAKES, "DIET" BARS AND OTHER NONSENSE

Plans that rely on the ingestion of special shakes, powders, bars or candies are among the biggest, most dastardly *scams* ever perpetrated on the American public. They are by far the most common, most well-known, and most profitable diet products in existence today. Included here are the products of many of the companies listed above, as well as products such as Ultra/Slim Fast, California Slim, Micro Diet, Pounds Off and many others.

All are based on a fundamentally *wrong,* but enticing premise: that short-term dieting can work... that eating shakes, powders or candy bars instead of meals in order to lose weight is safe, effective and permanent.

IT IS NOT.

These plans are all useless at best, outright harmful and dangerous at worst.

They are useless because they almost always fail to permanently accomplish their stated goals. Of course, they *are* seductive because there is almost always an immediate reduction of weight. But it's not difficult to lose some weight with a highly restrictive diet, especially in the beginning. Virtually *any* diet will do that for you. Water losses alone in the beginning of such diets often appear impressive (the water, of course, always comes back). What is difficult is keeping the weight off, and that is where all these diet programs fail miserably. In fact, it strongly appears that these plans *rely* on the fact that **almost everyone who becomes a customer will be back for more, because almost everyone will gain all their weight back.** What they seek, then, is built-in repeat business—paid in the coin of pain, disappointment, and poor health suffered by most of their clients.

Study after study has shown that more than 95% of these dieters ultimately fail. Almost no dieter achieves *permanent* weight control. And the reasons for this sorry state of affairs are very well understood by the companies selling the products that make it so. (BioSlim, not being a diet, *does* work, permanently.)

Perhaps the most callous, most outrageous example of how these companies operate is, in my opinion, the television commercial once aired by Ultra/Slim Fast in support of their very popular, very sugar-laden, nutritionally horrendous powdered diet product—wherein *salads*(!!) are attacked as *inferior diet food*(!!) as compared to their wonderful, synthetic cans of slop! Here is a truly mind-boggling display of irresponsible, misleading, *loathsome* advertising.

Do you really believe that weight loss by eating *shakes* or *candy bars* instead of real food can be healthful or permanent? Most people know this is not the case. But it's easy to fall into the trap: the goal is so strongly desired, the lure so enticing.

What we are talking about here is a never-ending cycle of wasted energy, health and money.

And, as if all this were not bad enough, some of these plans, particularly those that advocate drastic calorie restriction, can be positively dangerous: they have been known to cause gallstones, heart arrhythmias, sexual and menstrual dysfunction, and even *sudden death!*

In short: these products are *junk,* and should NEVER be used.

Avoid them completely, forever.

"MEAL REPLACEMENTS": TICKETS TO FAILURE

Here again, the products in question are produced by many of the companies investigated by the FTC for false and misleading claims (see above page 21).

Included are such organizations as:

- Jenny Craig, Inc.,
- Nutri/System Inc.,
- Diet Centers,
- Physicians Weight Loss Centers,
- Weight Watchers International,
- Micro Diet,

- and many others.

All of these programs produce artificially prepared pre-packaged "foods" for their clients to eat while "on the diet". All claim quick, easy, long-lasting weight loss, which, according to the FTC, are claims that are patently false and misleading.

As described under *Powders, Shakes and Other Nonsense* above, short-term, unnatural "diets" have been proven to be ineffective for long-term weight loss, and are potentially health-destructive.

In a sense, these programs—the ones that sell prepackaged, dehydrated, foil-wrapped, microwavable, nutritionally empty "meals" and "meal replacements"—are potentially *more* insidious than those selling the blatantly unnatural, synthetic garbage known as "diet powders", "diet shakes" or "diet bars". Most people know that "diet" powders, shakes and bars are for short-term use only. But the prepackaged meals are marketed as *permanent* alternatives to real food. People are advised to eat these "meals" for months, even *years*. This leads to nutritionally deficient users who routinely gain all their weight back, and more, as soon as they go back to eating any kind of normal diet.

These products are also mostly *junk*.

Avoid them!

"DESIGNER" DIETS: ATKINS, ET AL

One type of "designer diet" consists of specific foods that must be eaten to the exclusion of all others for a prescribed period of time. Usually the chosen foods, like *rice, grapefruit, watermelon* and others, are not individually unhealthful. It is, rather, the unnatural *restrictiveness* of the these diet types that make them unacceptable and potentially dangerous.

It is possible to lose weight with these programs. But because these plans are unnatural, unbalanced and generally unhealthful, as soon as a normal diet is reestablished all lost weight is almost certain to return.

Another category here is typified by the Atkins diet:

Be careful! The Atkins diet is seriously flawed, and can be quite dangerous. It consists of high fat foods, eaten virtually without restriction, heavily restricted carbohydrate intake and little attention to food quality and healthfulness. A state of *ketosis* is sought, even tested for with urine sticks to be sure the user has achieved it! "Ketosis" is the incomplete oxidation ("burning for energy") of fats resulting in the accumulation of intermediary (*acetyl-CoA*) molecules: it is an abnormal, undesirable, potentially dangerous state.

This diet can actually result in some weight loss. High fat foods taste good, and, since fats take longer to digest, people can feel full longer. These advantages, however, are **strongly** counterbalanced by the unhealthful effects of a high fat intake as well as by the dangers of inadequate nutrition this diet can create. (Sources: *A critique of low-carbohydrate ketogenic weight reduction regimens: A review of Dr. Atkins' Diet Revolution.* JAMA *224:1415-9, 1973; Dr. Atkins' Diet Revolution.* Med Lett *15(May 1):41-2, 1973*)

Potential side effects of the Atkins diet can include:
- Cognitive dysfunction (i.e., confusion, unclear thinking)
- Postural hypotension (low blood pressure and possibly dizziness with standing)
- Hyperlipidemia (high blood fat)
- High blood uric acid level (which can cause gout)
- Fatigue
- Irritability and tension
- Mood changes
- Glucose Intolerance
- Diarrhea
- Abnormal water losses due to ketosis
- Nutritional deficiencies (unless supplemented)
- Constipation
- Unusual food cravings

(Sources: *Friedman RB. Fad diets: Evaluation of five common types.* Postgrad Med *89(1):249-58, 1986; Morgan SL.*

Rational weight loss programs: A clinician's guide. J Am Coll Nutr 8(3):186-94, 1989)

In short: Stay **away** from this one!

Finally, there are diets with the words "X-Day Diet", where "X" equals some number of days, such as the 5, 6 or 7-Day Diets, et al. These are so ineffective, so *wrong* as to be ridiculous. Heavy dietary restrictions and meal replacements are followed by short periods of unrestricted eating. This will not work healthfully or permanently. Chances are these schemes will not work at all.

Once again, all these plans are strongly **not recommended**.

DRUGS

Most of these are stimulant compounds, and are too side-effect laden to recommend. The only over-the-counter (non-prescription) drug for which weight loss claims can legally be made is *phenylpropanolamine*, best known commercially as *Dexatrim* and *Acutrim*, which is actually a decongestant and a stimulant (a "sympathomimetic" in *medicalese*). Side effects may include dizziness, insomnia, heart palpitations, nervousness, and other unpleasantness.

A few of the newer prescription drugs, the best of which are *phentermine* (aka *Ionamin*) and now possibly *sibutramine* (aka *Meridia*), carry fewer side-effects than previously available drugs and can be quite effective. There *are* however, risks involved. Some of these drugs can cause *pulmonary hypertension*, a usually fatal disease, as well as heart rhythm and gastrointestinal disturbances, and other serious side-effects.

(Note: BioSlim *can* be done in combination with drug therapy, if desired and recommended by a physician. It is always best to stick to the more natural BioSlim plan, but sometimes, more rapid weight loss is necessary for medical or other reasons. The net effect of doing *both* BioSlim and drug therapy will be faster, permanent weight loss; BioSlim will remain once the drug(s) is stopped. Of course, this must be done under the supervision of a physician.)

In addition to the health risks, the problem with this (drugs-only) approach is that typically, *weight loss thus achieved cannot by its nature be permanent unless the drug is taken indefinitely.* Therefore, this method cannot be recommended unless it is used for a limited time under the care of a physician who knows you well and believes you need just a little help getting started on your program. The goal must be to wean you *off* the drug(s) as soon as possible.

A lifetime on medication certainly cannot, in good conscience, be deemed acceptable. The risks are very high.

There are far better, far *healthier* ways to go. Like BioSlim.

Trying to achieve permanent, healthful weight loss only through drugs, then, is <u>not recommended</u>.

SURGERY

"Stomach stapling" is the common term used to describe the surgery most often performed as treatment of obesity. There are others as well. All accomplish the same goals: either dramatically diminishing the size of the functional part of the stomach so that satiety is achieved with only a small amount of food, or diverting part(s) of the digestive process.

These are *very* drastic methods, and cannot be recommended to any but the most desperately ill, most hopeless cases. There are much, much safer and far more healthful ways to achieve the same ends. BioSlim.

Other methods such as liposuction and abdominal "tucks" fall under the category of cosmetic surgery and cannot be considered treatments of obesity. Their purpose is to improve the appearance of one or more isolated parts of the body. They in no way address the overall issue of weight control, and will not be discussed here further.

THE *ONLY* RIGHT WAY TO
HEALTHFUL, PERMANENT WEIGHT CONTROL

Fortunately, there *is* a way to accomplish healthful, permanent weight loss. It involves combining several complementary elements:

- **THE BIOSLIM FORMULAS:** See the *Nutrition: The Key to Health* and *The BioSlim Formulas* chapters below;
- **FOOD:** See *The BioSlim Food Plan* chapter below;
- **LIFESTYLE:** See the *Mastering Motivation* and *What To Do About Those Cravings* chapters below;
- **ACTIVITY:** See *The Activity Plan* chapter below and companion BioSlim book, *The BioSlim Activity Plan*.

In the following chapters, we will review what BioSlim is, how it came to be, and how all its elements work together to help you achieve your desired goals.

SIX

WHAT IS BIOSLIM?
ೠഔ

BioSlim is not a diet. "Dieting" is defined as: a program of calorie or fat gram counting done *temporarily* for the purpose of losing weight. Diets cannot work. BioSlim is instead simply an easy way to lose weight healthfully and *permanently*, a way to eat and a way to stay healthy. There is no calorie counting, no fat gram measurements and calculations and no total calorie restriction. Therefore, BioSlim is *not a diet* as that concept is commonly understood.

BioSlim is NOT meant to be used merely as a short-term way to lose weight, though that, too, can certainly be done effectively. But to use BioSlim as a quick-weight-loss tool is to lose the best part of the BioSlim concept: the idea that the achievement of good health and the maintenance of that health are *lifelong* issues. What sense does it make to turn one's life around, lose weight and start feeling good—only to go back to the same lifestyle that got you unhealthy and overweight in the first place?

This book, then, is not a "diet book" as the genre has come to be defined. It is, rather, about getting healthy and staying that way, with a special focus on losing weight. The weight loss achieved should be viewed as stemming naturally from the overall health gains realized, not just an end unto itself. In fact, viewing the weight loss achieved—though it may be rapid and rewarding right from the start—as the only goal of the BioSlim program is a strong invitation to failure later.

Don't, then, do this temporarily. Be prepared to *permanently* change your thinking about food and about health maintenance. Yes, you *can* lose weight very easily and quickly using the

BioSlim System (and with *Super BioSlim* as described in *Appendix*). It is easy to see how a "quick-fix" approach can be very tempting to someone who desperately wants to lose weight. But it is our purpose to help effect a *permanent* change in the reader's health and appearance. It would serve none of us well to have the intent of this book usurped for a purpose so much less than the one it was intended to serve.

DIETING FACTS

And if all these reasons are not enough to convince you to adopt BioSlim permanently, perhaps the following *Dieting Fact Review* will sway you.

DIETING FACT REVIEW

- Fully ninety-five percent (95%), or 19 out of 20 people who go on diets fail to reach their goals.

- Of the remaining 5%, approximately 80% (4% of the 5%) will *regain* the weight they lost (as do most of the original 95% who may lose some weight but never reach their goals).

- In many instances, **more weight is ultimately regained than was lost dieting**, caused by the reduction of metabolic rate that accompanies most "diets".

- It has now been clearly and scientifically proven that weight loss achieved through most forms of calorie restriction is virtually always **doomed to failure**. The human body responds to intermittent calorie restriction by learning to live with less calories—by **reducing metabolic rate!** Combined with the lean-body-weight (muscle mass) losses experienced by most dieters, which further reduce metabolic rate, this makes keeping weight off a <u>near-impossibility</u>.

- For many dieters, each successive diet makes it *more difficult* to keep the weight off, and more difficult to lose weight with the next diet.

- Many people today have reached the point where *any* food intake beyond a near-starvation diet causes weight gain. Does this sound familiar?

- Today's commercial weight loss programs take full advantage of these well-known facts. They continue to market their severely calorie-restricted diet schemes, using prepackaged, nutritionally empty foods, or worse—powdered "meal-replacements" or so-called "diet shakes" and "diet bars" that are supposed to substitute for one, two, and sometimes all three daily meals. It is difficult to believe that the companies marketing such schemes do not know that most of their customers today will be potential customers again tomorrow when they gain all their weight back (and then some). It would seem, in fact, that they not only know it, but *depend* on it as *part of their plan.*

- The use of pre-packaged, highly processed, dehydrated, unnatural, unhealthful, nutritionally empty and environmentally polluting "meals" or "meal substitutes" (Nutri/System, Jenny Craig, Diet Centers, Optifast, Medifast, Ultrafast, Micro Diet, and even Weight Watchers all use them, as do many others) can lead to more than just a failure to keep lost weight off. The risk of serious gallbladder, kidney, gastrointestinal, heart, metabolic and other diseases is believed to be significantly elevated in people undergoing rapid calorie-restriction-generated weight loss programs, particularly those using "meal substitutes" or "replacements".

- People whose weights continually fluctuate are at significantly higher risk of developing cardiovascular (heart and blood vessel) disease and diabetes than people who stay at stable weights, *even if those stable weights are at obese levels.* In other words, yo-yo dieting is itself a problem, even more so than simply being overweight.

Many of these points have been publicly announced by the Federal Trade Commission, which has already forced several companies in the diet industry to change their advertising claims in light of the ever-growing body of scientific data concerning the ineffective and harmful nature of their methods. (See above, beginning of this chapter.)

Had enough? If you are overweight, and/or tired all the time, in pain, sick too often, or otherwise unhealthy—you must accept the fact that *something* needs to change. What your specific "something" must be will become clear as you read on.

But it certainly *won't* lend itself to a thoughtless, quick fix. Problems fixed quickly, as we have seen, quickly lead right back to more of the same.

YOUR GOALS WITH BIOSLIM

1) WEIGHT LOSS. This is listed first because it's what BioSlim is about. Your weight loss may be rapid, up to eight or ten pounds in the first week, and anywhere from two to four or six pounds per week later on. Average weight loss is approximately two pounds per week. Some may lose only one pound in a week. Don't worry if you're in the lower ranges. Every one of us has his or her own internal schedule, based on the metabolic and biochemical individuality each of us possesses. It may even take a month or more to get going, and you may even need to look at *Super BioSlim* along the way—but if you follow the program as outlined, you *will* achieve your goals.

2) IMPROVEMENT IN ENERGY LEVEL. Most people report an improvement in stamina, concentration ability, and general energy level. This has to do with the elimination of harmful and/or allergenic foods from the diet, as well as with the increased use of health-building foods. And, importantly, the recommended all-natural BioSlim Formulas can do much to help support metabolic functions, particularly if the user has a history of nutritional deficiencies. They do much to add to the feeling of improvement in energy levels most people experience when they start the program.

3) IMPROVED APPETITE CONTROL. The combination of healthful foods, exercise, BioSlim Formulas and mood improvement leads to significant appetite reduction in most people on the BioSlim System. This is a major part of the effect BioSlim has on people, and is one of the more noticeable improvements people report.

4) MOOD IMPROVEMENT. Many people report that they feel happier and that their relationships are improved once they begin the program. There are many reasons for this effect, including: improved energy levels, weight loss, reversal of nutritional deficiencies, elimination of unhealthful, metabolically destructive foods, and the psychological boost many people feel when they start a program of self-improvement.

5) IMPROVED BOWEL HABITS. Though at first, some people may experience a change in bowel habits or some amount of intestinal gas, the vast majority of people on BioSlim report significant *improvements* in this area. Remember, a healthy bowel moves at least once daily, and even two or three times daily. The improvements seen on BioSlim stem from the all-natural BioSlim Formulas, the dietary changes, the increased water intake and the recommended activities.

6) FATTER POCKETBOOK. You will spend less on food because you'll be eating less empty, often expensive, nutritionally useless foods—and more of the health-building foods your body needs. You'll spend less on medical bills because you'll be both healthier and more self-sufficient when it comes to taking care of yourself. It has been estimated that if everyone in the United States, doctors and patients alike, practiced medicine and lived life using the preventive principles and methods described in this book, our yearly national expenditure on medical care could drop by *one-half* from its

current mind-numbing level of nearly about one *trillion* dollars.

7) GENERALLY IMPROVED HEALTH and "SIDE BENEFITS". If you follow the BioSlim program completely, you should experience greatly improved health. This statement can be made because BioSlim truly is a natural, *total* health system, designed not only to aid in weight loss, but with your *whole* body in mind. "Side benefits" are the counterparts to the "side effects" so common with drug-and-procedure-based treatments. Because BioSlim is a *natural* health system, using *no* drugs, your body can experience rewards and improvements in areas you never thought of.

The body *fixes itself,* given the opportunity to do so; BioSlim gives it the opportunity and support it needs to make that happen.

SEVEN

THE BEGINNING: WHY CHANGE IS ESSENTIAL
ଓଛଠ

BioSlim was born and raised in a medical office over a period of several years beginning in the summer of 1990. Prior to its release to the general public it went through years of gestation and clinical testing, nurtured then by the staff and patients of the Summa Medical Group, in Woodland Hills and Beverly Hills, California.

There were many, many people and events that led to the development of BioSlim. The process by which it all occurred illuminates much of what is troublesome in both the diet and medical establishments today, as well as what can be done about it. A quick review will help clarify what each of us can do to help ourselves and our families cope with these important issues, and why change is both necessary and inevitable.

BIOSLIM AND THE MEDICAL GROUP

The staff of Summa Medical Group committed itself to helping people find new, health-*enhancing* solutions to complement and improve upon today's crisis-based, drug-oriented approach to medicine—to finding the right *healthful* alternatives to what has become a dangerous and *un*healthy diet and weight loss industry.

For example: Drug therapy for human illness should always be kept to the *essential minimum.* You don't need an antibiotic every time you develop a sore throat or have a fever, but you do if you develop pneumonia. You don't need steroids every time your back or neck hurts or whenever you develop a rash, though you do if you suffer from adrenal insufficiency. And you certainly don't need tranquilizers and sleeping pills if you happen to feel nervous or anxious, or if you suffer from insomnia. There are other ways.

Have you ever wondered why almost every time you see your doctor, you get at least one prescription? Can you remember the last time you went to your doctor with a sore throat or a cold and *didn't* get an antibiotic? And has your child ever been to see a doctor with a cold or a sore ear and *not* gotten an antibiotic?

SUFFER THE CHILDREN

Our children, regrettably, bear the brunt of the worst part of the medical mishandling that affects so many of us today. Each new, ever more powerful oral antibiotic that is invented is usually used first on our children—the smallest, most defenseless members of society. Witness drugs like Augmentin, Suprax, Cipro, and many others. These are *enormously powerful* drugs that can and do wreak havoc in our children's bodies. And yet in many cases, these drugs and other medications are prescribed virtually indiscriminately. Incredibly, in some *seemingly* intractable cases of childhood illness, these or other powerful medications are prescribed as long-term *"prophylaxis"* ("prevention"), to be taken daily for months, sometimes *years*! As if nature made a mistake by not incorporating a little antibiotic pill dispenser in our children's digestive tracts!

The full story of what this kind of "therapy" does to a growing child's immune system and other body functions in the long run is still quite unknown. Moreover, recent studies have shown that the use of antibiotics in childhood often does nothing to forestall or control childhood illnesses. And yet the practice goes on virtually unabated!

The fact is, most experts in the specialty field of infectious disease agree that in most primary care cases (those diseases and patients who are treated in a general doctor's office, as opposed to in a hospital or by a specialist), it is best to use the <u>weakest</u> antibiotic that is likely to do the job required, not the strongest. The overuse of antibiotics by the medical establishment and by the meat industry (they are used on animals routinely) is directly responsible for much of the explosion of new, hyper-virulent strains of infectious organisms we are witnessing today, such as *tuberculosis, staphylococcus, streptococcus,* et al. The underlying problem is that micro-organisms (e.g., bacteria) multiply so rapidly that they quickly find ways—through their normal, natural evolution—to *resist* commonly used antibiotics. We are now, in fact, at the brink of a very serious worldwide health dilemma: the onslaught of new, highly antibiotic-resistant infectious diseases for which we literally have *no effective treatments.*

Despite all this, the chronic overuse—no, *ab*use—of antibiotics and many other drugs continues. And children continue to be among the prime targets of this abuse. The result is that the processes that lead to adult disease and chronic ill health often begin in childhood, and the way childhood diseases are treated by doctors today is one of the most dangerous parts of that process. Instead of throwing extremely powerful, potentially toxic drugs at our sick children, doctors should be talking to parents about:

- What kind of diet is the child eating?
- How much fluid does the child drink during the course of a typical day?
- How much milk and milk-containing food does the child consume each day? (Optimum = none! Milk-containing foods are linked to increased childhood infections and lung problems, such as asthma and bronchitis.)
- What is the state of the child's hygiene?
- Is the child unnecessarily exposed to other, contagious children or adults?
- What is the child's overall nutritional status?
- Is the child being fed or otherwise exposed to allergy-causing substances (e.g., milk, corn, airborne pollen, et al)

— a common cause of recurrent upper respiratory irritation and subsequent infection?
- Has the child been given sufficient replacement amounts of the normal, friendly, health-maintaining bacteria that are destroyed by each successive course of antibiotics?
- If the child is breast-feeding, is the *mother* taking adequate care of her own nutritional needs, and is *she* avoiding potentially harmful drugs and foods?

How many times have you been asked about these issues at your doctor's office? If you're like most people, the answer is probably zero, or nearly zero. Perhaps it is time, then, to think about finding a physician who is concerned with just such issues—one who *worries* about using powerful medications on little children. You would be hard-pressed to find anything more important you can do to help improve the current and future health of your child.

Now, to understand how BioSlim came to be, let's follow the story of our children as they grow.

WHAT HAPPENS AS THE CHILD GROWS: THE FREQUENT INEVITABILITY OF OBESITY

After surviving recurrent childhood illnesses, which eventually stop only when he or she grows too old to continue having them, our child enters young adulthood. When adolescents or teenagers get sick, they usually receive the same kind of treatment they got as children, though perhaps from different doctors. There continues to be little or no attention paid to diet and health maintenance.

Luckily, the importance of a proper activity level has now been generally recognized to the point where most people are now at least *aware* of its desirability, though many still don't act on that awareness. Education on nutrition and appropriate food choices, though, is generally left to parents and peers, with little or no input from the medical community.

Parents, though, are often completely unaware of the realities of modern nutrition. As a result, the nutritional education our growing young adult gets at home is generally either non-existent or completely erroneous.

And what is our teenager likely to learn about nutrition and health from his or her peers? Among most of today's young people, good nutrition means: cheeseburgers, french fries and pizza, washed down with cola drinks, topped off with ice cream. At home, the day's major food ingestion ends at dinner, which usually consists of fat-laden meat, fried food dripping with oil, possibly a small salad drowned in oily salad dressing, and a dessert of pie topped with whipped cream. A late-night snack may follow, the nutritional characteristics of which are similarly horrendous.

There's more. One recent study found that *television viewing* is directly related to reduction of metabolic rate in children and leads to obesity (possibly due to decreased physical activity). And we all know how much time our children spend sitting in front of the television.

And so it goes. Often the child is obese by the age of 6 or 7 years, sometimes sooner. If the *child* manages to escape this fate — sooner or later the *adult* becomes fat. In any event, obesity in many such cases is virtually unavoidable. The child, the teenager, and certainly the adult never have a chance.

The fact is: Most of the food eaten by most people in the "developed" world today cannot adequately nourish human beings. The so-called "Western diet" will nearly *always* lead to ill-health and obesity, sooner or later. Some people, through life-long starvation diets or through aggressive exercise programs, or through the sheer luck of being born with robust metabolisms, can continue on this kind of diet and avoid obesity through early middle age. But eventually, if one lives long enough, obesity will almost *inevitably* set in under these circumstances, unless significant changes are made.

* * *

It has been estimated that the *"average"* adult gains one to two pounds per year. At that rate, this "average" adult is obese by the age of 40-45 years. Amazingly, and sadly, the overweight state is now considered the de facto norm for older adults by many authorities. In other words, more people who are past the age of 40 in Western society are overweight than not, once the age factor is eliminated from the calculation of what is "overweight".

Making obesity "normal" with increasing age makes no sense; and gaining weight with age should *not* be considered inevitable or acceptable just because it happens to so many people. It is still unhealthful, and is considered "normal" only because so many people are abnormal in this way that their numbers change the statistical analysis that determines what is normal in the first place.

NOTE: One lesson to be learned from this is simply a further corroboration of what was discussed earlier: don't look to weight charts and tables to gauge your health or your progress—look in the mirror.

Next, we'll review *how* the "typical Western diet" impacts your health and your weight.

WHAT IS RIGHT AND WHAT IS WRONG WITH THE WAY WE EAT — AND WHAT TO DO ABOUT IT

There are, broadly speaking, three major problems with the typical Western diet:

I) There is an enormous amount of insubstantial, nutritionally empty—or worse, nutritionally *harmful*—food available today. These foods are packaged by giant food companies to be highly attractive and delicious. The problem is that too many of these foods are so unnatural, so devoid of those elements that human beings need to survive, that the term "food" cannot be rightfully applied to them. A better term would be *"junk"*, or even *"toxic waste"*. Call it anything... but it's not "food".

Here are some examples of common *non-foods* that nevertheless pass for "food". Ideas for healthful and delicious alternatives to many of these items are discussed later in this book and in the companion *BioSlim CookBook*.

- Margarine
- Oily salad dressings
- Potato chips
- All chips made with oil
- Ice cream
- Mayonnaise
- Cream cheese
- Sugar (white table)
- White flour
- Candies
- Most oils
- Soft drinks
- French fries
- Most breakfast cereals (if made with sugar, oil, or white flour)
- And many more

Now, we've all eaten some, if not all, of these items at one time or another. That doesn't make it right or healthful. It does, however, reveal how we are all subject to tastes developed in infancy and childhood, and to peer and social pressures to conform to the *eating norm*. In youth, we tend to eat whatever is given us. As we grow, we learn to enjoy those foods to which we have most frequently been exposed.

But this phenomenon cuts both ways: many's the time I've heard from my patients how their children just *love* eating green vegetables, or whole grain breads, and even *spirulina,* an extremely nutritious food that can dramatically improve one's nutritional well-being—but which has a less-than-wonderful flavor. Despite the "terrible" taste, some children grow up *loving* it. Case in point: my own two children, who *ask* for their spirulina—because they like it so much. (And they are *so* cute drinking it from their bottles!)

It's all a matter of taste, for which, proverbially, there is no accounting. "Taste" is an acquired sense, molded largely by childhood experience.

II) There is too much food! We are blessed in the U.S. with an abundance of just about everything, especially food. And most food, particularly the least healthful choices such as white flour products and other highly processed food, is not very expensive: most people can obtain far more food than their bodies need. This abundance of choice is itself a potential source of trouble, for it makes resisting temptation difficult. It also makes selecting the good from the bad a formidable task.

The solution lies in sticking to basic principles—such as the BioSlim Principles outlined later in this book. Choosing right from wrong can become simple—almost second nature—once the underlying concepts are clarified and accepted.

III) Americans generally eat an *unbalanced* diet of too many carbohydrates, too little protein, too much fat. High-carbohydrate foods are the ones made from flour and sugars; high-protein foods are the meats, poultry, fish, eggs, milk and soy products (and spirulina!); fats are the fats in food, and oil.

The optimal diet should consist of an approximate balance of carbohydrates to proteins, and NO ADDED FATS! In other words, balance the amount of carbs to protein by either weight, volume or the eyeball test (*look* at it!), and avoid all fats and oils that are *added* to any food (as opposed to the naturally occurring fats and oils found in many foods).

The improper balance of these food elements leads to insulin derangement in the body, among other things, and a higher rate of body fat storage. In short, it will exacerbate obesity. For more on this, see Chapters 3 *(Why Do We Become Overweight")* and 11 (*The Food Plan)*.

There is much that is healthful and nutritious alongside all the available junk food. Within our general abundance is an assortment of whole, natural food such as has never before been so readily available. It is not necessary to buy and eat white bread: there are whole grain products galore to choose from. It is not necessary to buy and eat prepackaged, dehydrated, overprocessed, nutritionally empty foods: you can instead choose from a fabulous array of real, *recognizable,* whole foods—foods that nature intended humans to consume and to be nourished by.

The choice between good, health-*building* food and empty, health-*destroying* food is <u>*yours*</u>*! You* must decide to make the change—and you must do it in a way that satisfies you and makes you happy if you are to continue with your new, healthful food plan.

In the next section, we'll start the process of helping you get in shape *permanently.* But first, let's examine what happens when the nearly-inevitable eventually occurs: when your scale keeps going up and up, and suddenly, it's obvious to you that you've become *heavy.*

What will be your likely reaction?

EIGHT

WHEN THE SCALE ALWAYS RISES: COMMON REACTIONS
☙☙

Now that we have explored the virtual inevitability of obesity for the "average" person eating the "average" Western diet, let's examine what most overweight people *do* when this problem occurs. Typically, people's reactions fall into three broad categories:

1) Those who never bother to try to lose weight. We call this the *"Who cares?"* group.

2) Those who are continually trying to lose weight. Women tend to fall into this category more commonly than men. These folks are always "going on a diet", always hungry, always fighting to keep their weight down. Sound familiar? This unfortunate state is *very* common today. We call it the *"Hopelessly hungry"* syndrome.

3) Those who try dieting a few times only to give up, convinced that the overweight state is simply unavoidable. We call this the *"Oh, well, I tried..."* group.

"WHO CARES?"

People in this category may believe that obesity is *"In my genes"*, or *"It can't be helped—it's my metabolism"*. Some truly and simply don't care. Most often, though, people care very much, but hide their concerns behind psychologically formidable barricades of excuses and ill-defined motivations.

Some in this category derive a level of *"secondary gain"* from being overweight. "Secondary gain" is another way of saying: "ulterior motive"—actions taken for reasons other than the motivations claimed. Being overweight *can* have its rewards, however unfulfilling and specious. While these rewards are often more perceived than real, it is each individual's *perception* of reality that is most important and motivating to that individual. We act on our own understanding of reality, not anyone else's.

Some examples of "rewards" gained by remaining overweight are:

- There is less perceived need to take responsibility for personal attractiveness.
- Sympathy from friends and family members may be more forthcoming.
- An underlying feeling of low self-esteem and poor self-worth, if present, can be justified or reinforced.
- There is a built-in excuse for failure. Obesity can provide easy excuses: "I failed because I'm fat→ my being fat is not my fault→ therefore my failure is not my fault." This kind of thinking can be repeated over and over—as often as necessary.
- For some, anxiety and fear are overcome with food.
- Depression may be drowned in an ocean of food.
- There may be less perceived need to worry about finding and keeping a mate.
- Once a mate is found, obesity can be used as a means of minimizing intimacy.
- The underlying need many people have to self-destruct can be fulfilled.

THE SELF-DESTRUCTIVE IMPULSE

Why is it that so many of us do so much that is harmful to ourselves? What is this rarely-discussed aspect of human nature that for many lies hidden at the center of core beliefs and motivations — the impulse to self-destruct? Where it stems from is not well understood, and not often contemplated. But that it exists is very clear.

Why else do we so often do so much that is obviously harmful to our own security and well-being? Why do we live in polluted cities, smoke cigarettes, play with guns, go to war, build nuclear weapons, eat junk food, ignore our families, work too hard, rest too little, break laws, gamble, have Hitlers and Stalins in the world, pollute the environment in which we must live, and continually ignore our spiritual side?

Collectively as a world-wide society, nationally as Americans, and personally as individuals struggling to survive on this planet, we each of us, from time to time, take actions that can only be explained as self-destructive.

Why?

Perhaps it is the knowledge of mortality that each of us carries. We don't often allow ourselves to fully accept this. People *talk* about mortality, but only rarely fully accept it as inevitable reality. We tend to think of it as something that happens to people in movies, to older people, to sick people, to unlucky people. To *other* people. Never to ourselves. But at the center of our hearts and minds lies the truth that is often not bearable. And so, the self-destructive impulse is born—out of frustration and a sense of hopelessness. Out of a futile attempt to prove false that which we know to be true; to show ourselves and the Universe that it ain't so!—that we *can* risk life and limb and survive—that we are, in fact, immortal, despite all evidence to the contrary.

And so we have doctors and nurses outside intensive care units smoking cigarettes by the fistful while joking about the poor guy inside on a respirator dying of lung cancer; and doctors prescribing drugs, radiation, and all manner of dangerous procedures—instead of health, nutrition and disease prevention; and people subsisting their whole lives on junk food and convincing themselves that yes, it's OK to be fat.

THE "HOPELESSLY HUNGRY" SYNDROME

An enormous number of people fall into this category. The entire multi-*billion* dollar diet industry exists mostly because of them.

> **FACT:** Fully 95%, or *19 out of every 20* people who go on a diet, fail to fully reach their goals! They, and most of the remaining 5%, will eventually regain all their lost weight. Only approximately ONE PERCENT of all dieters will achieve their goals *permanently*. This, more than any other, is an incredible statistic—one worth contemplating.

Most people who have ever felt the need to lose weight have experienced this reaction. It's the can-do, "I'm going to lick this thing" attitude that *usually* gets things done.

But not when it comes to dieting.

Since diets don't work, this can-do approach is fundamentally doomed to failure. It's the *tools* used that fail, not the underlying motivation. Without the right tools, virtually anyone who "goes on a diet" is destined to remain "hopelessly hungry".

If you recognize yourself as being in this category—and most overweight people do—take heart! BioSlim is *terrific* at helping people just like you achieve their previously elusive goals. Promise yourself you will never, ever again fall into the diet trap — you know, the one the diet industry assumes you are already in. "Dieting", defined as a temporary measure of calorie and/or fat gram counting and food quantity restriction, is useless and hopeless at best, outright harmful at worst. (See *Your Choices: Weight Control Review* above for a review of the problems associated with a variety of common weight loss methods.)

"OH WELL, I TRIED..."

People in this category fall somewhere between categories 1 and 2. They have tried and failed and given up. And no wonder — it's not easy trying to lose weight permanently on the typical

Western diet, or with the commercially available diet programs. Practically, the only way to do it is to go hungry for a long time... until the weight comes off. But unless the dieter is prepared to face a *lifetime* of hunger, weight lost through this kind of deprivation will almost certainly return, often with a little extra poundage as "interest on the loan".

Remember, "going on a diet" does not work! We have previously examined all the confusion and *dys*information surrounding the issue of weight loss. We have shown how this confusion feeds the coffers of a multi-billion dollar industry, and how the unsuspecting, poorly-informed dieting consumer pays the price for this confusion in a never-ending cycle of wasted energy, health and money. In view of all this, is it any wonder that there are so many people in the *"Oh well, I tried..."* category?

The issues that motivate this group typically combine those from *both* of the preceding two. Sometimes, the individual may simply be more easy-going, less anxious, and less concerned about personal appearance than others. Others borrow heavily from the *"Who cares?"* group: they seem to try to straighten out their health and weight, at least half-heartedly, only to give up quickly upon first failure. It's easier to give up (*"Who cares?"*) when you can say *"Oh well, I tried..."*.

Still others have faithfully gone through a *"Hopelessly hungry"* phase only to find it truly hopeless. They too eventually end up saying *"Oh well, I tried"*.

REVIEW of WEIGHT REACTION CATEGORIES

It should be noted here that these three categories are, naturally, not written in stone—they are meant merely as general tools to help in the understanding of what motivates different people to act in certain ways. Each individual is guided by issues and concepts far too numerous and complex to categorize neatly in any book. So if you're trying to figure out which category you fall into, keep in mind that you are likely to find truth and relevance in *more than one category*—usually in some combination of *all* of them.

Life is rarely simple.

Each of these ways of dealing with excessive weight carries with it a number of problems. None holds the promise of truly solving the dieting dilemma. None will work in the long run. None is conducive to good health.

But whichever category most closely matches yours, take heart — and read on! You *will* succeed this time! The BioSlim System you are now discovering can and will change your life. Once absorbed, you will find BioSlim's concepts and recommendations so logical, so *sensible* that following them will soon become second nature.

And best of all: they work!

SOLUTIONS

We have reviewed the problems. Solutions lay in the pages ahead. They depend on a full understanding of the basic problems, one of which is that most people in Western society eat so little food that contains any worthwhile nutrition whatsoever that ill-health and excess poundage is virtually inevitable.

If you are overweight and reading this book in the expectation of finally discovering a way to lose your extra weight permanently, *please:* be prepared to adopt some new concepts about the food you eat; how, when and in what balance you eat it; and the BioSlim System in general, including the powerful and important BioSlim Formulas. With that, you will soon find the BioSlim system so easy to follow, so fulfilling, enjoyable, and most important, *healthful*—your ultimate success will be assured!

NINE

THE BEST, MOST HEALTHFUL WAY TO ACHIEVE YOUR OPTIMAL WEIGHT
ೞ⃝

The BioSlim program represents the only safe, healthful way to lose weight. This may seem like a difficult statement to support, but it is, in fact, completely true.

BioSlim is not a new weight loss fad, nor a gimmick by which to achieve quick, easy, temporary weight reduction. BioSlim is, rather, a straightforward, easy-to-follow, entirely sensible and logical system whereby anyone can lose excess weight and achieve better health in the process. Many people who have followed the BioSlim program for weight loss have also reported significant, often dramatic improvements in long-standing health problems that had previously either gone untreated or were treated ineffectively. Even serious illnesses such as high blood pressure, diabetes mellitus, asthma, and certain cardiovascular diseases can be improved once the BioSlim program is adopted.

The reason all these *side-benefits* can occur is that BioSlim embraces a way of life that is far more in tune with what nature intended for our bodies than the typical Western lifestyle and eating pattern. We live in a world full of humankind's perversions of nature. Everything from pollution to processed food to radiation exposure to atmospheric ozone depletion. Among the worst of all is the explosive growth of the use of drugs as the preferred, often *only* method for treating most human ailments.

There is an enormous conceit evident in the way we as a species ignore nature's intentions, twist the natural order of things to our convenience, and believe that we can tinker with our bodies using toxic chemicals (e.g., drugs) and somehow achieve a positive result. BioSlim represents a step in the direction of sanity; a step toward that which is natural and *good* for our bodies, and *away* from the disease and disfigurement that big business and big medicine so avidly promote.

You *can* do it. Everything changes sooner or later.

And the *world* is changed one small step at a time.

If enough people tune out the confusion, the cynicism, the deceit... it *will* change. Just as the accumulated business decisions of many unrelated concerns have led to the current state of the American diet and health care systems, so can a new movement begin as each of us, individually, does what he or she must. Taken together, our actions can and will create a new paradigm.

Everything changes.

STAYING HAPPY: VITAL TO SUCCESS

No one is *forced* to eat the non-food, processed junk that so pervades our lives. In the BioSlim program, you will see how you can make the *right choices*—the ones that will make you healthier and *lengthen your life*—**without making you feel deprived or unhappy in any way**.

This last is one of BioSlim's primary goals: to create a system that you—yes *you, personally*—can live with and *be happy with*. That is the only way to make sure you continue your healthful new ways for the rest of your (longer!) life.

Anything you do that you're not happy with—such as "going on a diet", or starving yourself—**you will one day stop!** Nothing could be more obvious, right? Anyone doing something unpleasant will not, given a choice, continue doing it indefinitely. Only by creating a uniquely personal program *for yourself*—using the guidance and information the BioSlim program provides—and making it fit *your* needs and desires so that *you're* happy with it, can you achieve permanent improvement.

In the following chapters we will explore ways for you to accomplish *all* your goals—safely, healthfully, and permanently.

SECTION TWO

THE BIOSLIM PRINCIPLES

MEDICAL CONSIDERATIONS

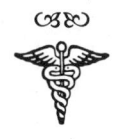

BioSlim was designed to be appropriate for everyone. Indeed, there is no one who, under normal conditions, cannot safely go on this program. There *are,* though, circumstances that require special attention and there are certain disease states that require a doctor's attention prior to embarking on any change of diet and lifestyle. Prudence dictates that everyone should check with the health care practitioner who knows him or her best before starting a program of weight loss or increased activity. Certainly, if you have ANY illness that requires medication or the supervision of a health professional, check with your doctor before starting a weight loss program.

If the doctor disapproves, though, be sure to ask *why.* Unfortunately, many doctors are so locked into their "drugs and surgery" approach to "health" that they will reject *any* more natural, more sensible approach out of hand, for no logical reason that they can quantify. Therefore, always ask *why.* And by the way, that same rule applies to *anything* your doctor, or anyone, else tells you to do. You should always seek to understand as best you can any advice that aims to change in any way the state of your health and life. And you must *keep* asking questions until you understand everything to your satisfaction.

Your health is and must always be *your* responsibility, not your doctor's. Never give up control. Always be involved, and always seek to understand what is happening to you. That is the best health insurance you can get.

Take charge of your own body! And remember: your physician should respond to your positive attitude about your health. If not, find one that will. They are out there; you just have to be clear about what you want, then go out and get it!

TEN THINGS TO SAY TO YOUR DOCTOR TO HELP IMPROVE YOUR HEALTH

1) I want to get well, but I also want to *stay* well. How do I accomplish this?
2) Please don't give me any drugs to take unless it is truly necessary. I do not come to you expecting miracles every time. If I can heal naturally, let's do it that way.
3) My symptoms are certainly disturbing to me, but I am more concerned with why I got sick in the first place and how I can prevent it from recurring.
4) What dietary suggestions can you make that might help with my problem and with my general health?
5) I've been going through a lot of stress. What bearing, if any, does that have on my current problem? What can I do to reduce my stress level?
6) Are these tests necessary? Why? Are there any dangers or side-effects from these tests?
7) Please explain these lab results to me so that I may understand what's going on in my body.
8) May I call you or your staff if I have any questions later?
9) I know I have a specific problem right now, but what about my general health? How can I improve it and how can I stay generally healthy?
10) I'm ready to accept any reasonable advice you may have about how I can change my lifestyle, my diet, my general nutrition and my social life to achieve better health.

TEN WARNING SIGNS TO WATCH FOR IN YOUR DOCTOR

1) The doctor appears unhealthy—obesity, a smoking habit, and drug, chemical or alcohol dependencies are examples of easily identified problems.
2) The doctor speaks curtly, avoids eye contact, and gives only cursory explanations of what he or she is doing, planning, and thinking about your case; he or she is distracted or has a hurried manner.
3) "Your diet is not important — just eat the four basic food groups and you'll have nothing to worry about."
4) "It's all in your head, dear."
5) "Take these pills and everything will be OK."
6) "Don't worry about your general health — let's just take care of your current problem."
7) "Stress has nothing to do with your problems."
8) "You don't need to understand these laboratory tests."
9) "Taking a vitamin or nutritional supplement is always stupid; don't waste your time and money."
10) "We can't take any telephone questions—we're just too busy."

* * *

We will now review common diseases and conditions and their interactions with the BioSlim System. The advice given here should not be considered a substitute for the attention of your physician, but rather as an aid to understanding these disorders and how to best help yourself by improving diet and lifestyle. In each case, we will describe the condition, discuss how it is recognized and treated, address how the BioSlim program interacts with it, and review the nutritional factors most important to that condition. Details on individual nutrients—what they are, their effect on the human body, and where they can best be obtained—may be found in the *"Nutrition: The Key To Health"* chapter below.

Note: there are no medications known to conflict significantly with BioSlim.

The following is a review, in alphabetic order, of common individual diseases and disorders.

♦ ADRENAL GLAND DYSFUNCTION

The adrenal glands lie over the kidneys, one on each side of the body. Their purpose includes the production of many important hormones that control such important body functions as mineral balance, blood pressure, kidney function, sex hormone function, blood sugar, and the response to stress, among others.

There are many disorders of the adrenals which we cannot address here, but there are two that are notable in that they are more common than the others and in that they can powerfully impact weight and energy levels. The first is *adrenal cortical insufficiency.* Symptoms are often non-specific and vague, which is why this diagnosis is often missed by primary care physicians. They include: fatigue, weakness, weight loss, low blood pressure, nausea and non-specific abdominal pain. Someimes, there are areas of skin darkening. If you have these symptoms, you should be checked for this syndrome by a physician. Treatment (typically hormone replacement) is usually highly effective.

A second adrenal disorder is called *Cushing's syndrome,* a condition of *too much* adrenal hormone production. Symptoms include: weight *gain,* particularly in the middle part of the body, high blood sugar or sugar intolerance, muscle weakness, easy bruisability, muscle weakness, and many others. Each of these symptoms can be caused individually by many other factors. But if you have several of them simultaneously, you should be checked by your physician. This is a serious but treatable disorder.

While these ailments in their full-blown states are indeed serious, there are people who suffer from *mild* adrenal insufficiency, making them chronically fatigued and sickly, without actually endangering their lives.

If you have received a clean bill of health from your doctor, and require no specific treatment, yet suffer from some of the symptoms listed here, you should follow the BioSlim program very closely. It is designed, through its diet and activity plans and with the aid of the many adrenal-supportive nutrients in the BioSlim Formulas, to help your body normalize its functions, and to help improve your sense of well-being.

◆ AGING

Here is one disease we are all going to get one day. So far, it seems inevitable. But is there something you can do now to slow it down? Can you forestall the ravages of old age somehow?

The answer is: yes! There is much that can be done. First and foremost: *get healthy!* Healthy bodies live longer and better. To accomplish this, you must achieve a weight level that is healthy *for your body*, and you must make sure you are receiving all the nutrients your body needs, to the best of current nutritional knowledge.

The best way to achieve all this? BioSlim! Your weight will normalize, and all your nutritional needs are well covered.

There are some particular nutrients that are useful in helping diminish or forestall the effects of aging. These are called "*antioxidants*". Their function is to diminish the damaging effects of certain chemical processes that are continually going on in your body. If concepts like "free radical scavenging" may be a bit too esoteric to cover in detail here, it is nevertheless important to note that the overall effect of these nutrients is to diminish the cellular and sub-cellular damage that accumulates over time in your body.

Now where can you get a good supply of antioxidants? Well, you already have it—in the BioSlim Formulas! They contain the most important, vital and protective antioxidants, including selenium, vitamin E, vitamin C, and a variety of antioxidant-containing plant extracts.

Of course, if you smoke or are exposed to any dangerous chemicals, and you are concerned about slowing down your aging process—stop these activities and exposures immediately! All the antioxidants in the world will not protect your body from that kind of assault on its health and proper function.

It is worth mentioning one other fact regarding slowing down the aging clock: **Many studies have shown, quite conclusively, that *lowering* overall food consumption will *lengthen* healthy productive life.** The less you eat, the longer you'll live, healthfully.

Way it is, folks.

♦ ALLERGIES AND SUBSTANCE SENSITIVITIES

Allergies to all kinds of substances are *very* common. You name it, and there is somebody, somewhere allergic to it. There are people who are allergic to tap water and *air!*

Sensitivity to food is an area of some controversy in medicine. But there is no question that it exists. If you suffer from food sensitivities, you'll be happy to note that BioSlim intrinsically avoids many of the most common allergenic foods — simply by avoiding highly processed, chemical-laden items. But it is possible to be allergic to *good* food too. If, by some unlucky chance, you happen to be allergic to one of the healthful foods recommended in the BioSlim Food Plan, or to a nutritional supplement, you may have to cut it out.

If you feel you may be allergic or sensitive to any food or food supplement, the only way to find out for sure is to stop ingesting the suspected item for at least 3-4 days, see if your symptoms disappear, then *restart* taking in the suspected product to see if symptoms return. If they do, you should *repeat* the test to see if the symptoms return again, and if they are lessened or increased the second time around. If they are milder, you can continue to use the product, with care. If they are worse, you may have to stop. This method of *avoidance* followed by *challenge* is the most accurate way—often better than any medical test—to determine the presence or absence of allergy/sensitivity to food, and for that matter, to just about anything.

The medical treatment of allergies often consists of avoidance (see above), desensitization (done by a physician), and/or symptom reduction with medication.

NUTRITIONAL FACTORS: Respiratory allergies may be helped by vitamin A. General allergies often respond to pantothenic acid, the other B-vitamins, vitamin C, bioflavonoids, vitamin E, calcium, and especially magnesium. Also found useful is the herb *Stinging Nettle*. Note that the BioSlim Formulas contain a carefully tested balance of all of the nutrients listed here in their correct quantities.

♦ ANEMIA

Anemia is a condition of too few red blood cells or too little hemoglobin in the bloodstream. These elements are responsible for *cellular respiration,* which literally means "the breathing of cells". Each cell in your body requires a continuous supply of oxygen, which is supplied to it by the bloodstream, carried by the red blood cells. When this supply runs low, your body cannot function properly. Symptoms may include: fatigue, dizziness, generalized weakness, pallor, insomnia, abdominal pain, loss of appetite, dry skin, brittle nails, heart trouble, confusion or loss of concentration ability, and many others.

Anemia can be caused by a variety of factors, including a deficiency of the mineral *iron*, hypothyroidism (a thyroid hormone deficiency, discussed below), recurrent or chronic disease of any kind, certain diseases of the bone marrow, peptic ulcers, and many other, less common ailments, including some inherited ones.

Iron deficiency, by far the most common cause of anemia, is most often found in women prior to menopause due to the monthly loss of blood. It can, of course, also be caused by abnormal conditions such as those affecting the spleen or internal bleeding from ulcers, tumors, etc.

Remember when testing for iron levels not to ingest any food, iron or multi-nutrient supplement in the 12-14 hours prior to the test. This is not necessary for the direct tests for anemia that measure the amount of red cells present (called *hematocrit*, *hemoglobin* and *red cell count*).

Besides iron, there are other nutritional deficiencies that can lead to anemia, including those of vitamin B12 (common in vegetarians), folic acid, the mineral copper, vitamin B6, vitamin C and vitamin E. Deficiencies of vitamin B1, vitamin B2, pantothenic acid or niacin may in turn cause a reduced absorption of iron and may lead to an iron-deficiency anemia.

Anemia is a very common disorder. If you suffer from the symptoms described, you should be checked by a physician to be sure you don't have any of the more serious causes of this ailment.

NUTRITIONAL FACTORS: If you have a clean bill of health from your doctor, you should address the nutritional deficiencies that are probably causing your problem. Make sure you get enough iron: the best way is take an iron supplement, or use the BioSlim Vita/Min Formula, which, taken in full doses, contains sufficient iron for most purposes. In severe cases of iron deficiency, additional iron should be taken. Don't overdo it, though. Too much iron can cause problems too.

Note: Keep all iron-containing pills out of reach of children!

And don't forget the other important nutrients your body must have in order to keep you supplied with enough red blood cells. These nutrients are all also present, in correct balance, in the BioSlim Formulas.

♦ ARTHRITIS

Arthritis is defined as "joint inflammation". Symptoms include pain, swelling, heat and/or redness of and around any joint of the body. Any one of these symptoms is sufficient to make the diagnosis, though they may all be present simultaneously.

There are many esoteric forms of arthritis, but only two common ones: *osteoarthritis* and *rheumatoid arthritis.* Osteoarthritis, also called "degenerative joint disease", is just that: a disease where the internal structure of the joint degenerates, causing excessive friction, swelling, deformity, and pain. It most often affects the large joints of the hips and knees, as well as the much-used joints of the hands.

Rheumatoid arthritis is a more generalized, more serious ailment, and is one of a group known as the *"autoimmune disorders".* It is believed to be caused mostly by the body's own immune system "going haywire" and attacking parts of the joints as if they were foreign invaders (like viruses or bacteria). This condition can cause far more harm in the body than joint destruction and pain, including, among others, heart and lung nodules, severe fatigue, anemia, white blood cell abnormalities and kidney problems. Commonly though, symptoms and signs are limited to the joints.

Symptoms of rheumatoid arthritis are chronic joint pain, swelling and inflammation, most often of the joints closest to the palms of the hands, and most severely felt in the mornings.

Both these forms of arthritis should be diagnosed and followed by a physician.

NUTRITIONAL FACTORS: There are many exciting new findings in this area. Rheumatoid arthritis sufferers should *avoid* the following foods: tomato, potato, eggplant, peppers (all kinds: bell, chili, the black kind used as a spice, red pepper, etc.), tobacco in all its forms, and all milk products. All but milk are members of the *Nightshade* group of foods, which can exacerbate the symptoms of some rheumatoid arthritis sufferers. There may be other foods that exacerbate symptoms in certain individuals. Experimentation with and elimination of those foods is encouraged.

SUPPLEMENTATION that may be helpful in arthritis: vitamin C, bioflavonoids (such as *quercetin*), vitamin B6, and GLA, one of the Essential Fatty Acids. All but the GLA are found in balanced doses in the BioSlim Formulas. GLA is available in gelcaps, and should be taken by anyone suffering from arthritis. On a more experimental level, SOD (SuperOxide Dismutase) and apple cider vinegar may be helpful.

CASE HISTORY: Angie is a 50 year old woman who came in as a new patient, and proceeded to describe her symptoms over the past year: debilitating fatigue, foot pain in the mornings which later progressed to foot and hand pains, and wrist pain. Angie works as a legal secretary, and uses her hands to type all day long at work. I suspected carpal tunnel syndrome, but decided to check for rheumatoid arthritis as well (her grandfather had had "some kind of arthritis").

Angie's labs revealed a raging case of rheumatoid arthritis. We assumed that the rheumatoid condition had also caused a mild carpal tunnel syndrome, a possible complication involving the wrist joints.

Angie started on a strict dietary program, avoiding all nightshades and milk-containing products. Since she was a smoker, she was told that she *must* quit (we do that—use the word *must*—where there is significant disease present). A complete nutritional program was begun, as outlined above.

Her symptoms abated over the next four to six weeks and she is now symptom-free, except occasionally on a morning following a day of "cheating".

♦ **ASTHMA**
See LUNG DISORDERS.

♦ **BACK PAIN**
This is the most common cause of lost worker time in the U.S. today. There are many causes for it, including serious spinal column disorders, but the most common is low back strain.

Due to the unique and rather unwieldy way human beings walk around, there are tremendous pressures that can build up in the area of the lower back. *Sitting* is the position most problematic for anyone suffering from low back strain, particularly sitting in a position where the knees are *lower* than the hips; the worst example is the driving position, where the legs are extended downward and outward from the body.

Medical treatment consists of rest followed by special therapeutic exercises and sometimes, drugs. As always, you should strive to get through your problem without having to resort to drugs. Note that your physician is not usually a good source for therapeutic exercises. Try a *good* chiropractor ("good" is defined here as spending more than two minutes per visit with you—at least 15–20 minutes is needed for proper, personal attention—and as *not* "cracking" except in the most gentle, controlled way.) Also, see the *BioSlim Activity Plan* book for many good ideas, such as the wonderful *Hip-Psoas-Calf Stretch*, which helps in many cases, and the other positions and stretches in the *Back and Hips* and *Problem Solving* sections of that book.

NUTRITIONAL FACTORS: See under ARTHRITIS.

♦ CANCER

In cancer, certain cells grow uncontrollably in the body. We cannot hope to cover the vastness of this subject in this book. We will limit our discussion to nutritional and preventive aspects, leaving matters of diagnosis and treatment to the personal physician under whose care anyone with this disease should be.

It is worth noting, though, that what passes for "treatment" of most forms of cancer is euphemistically named at best. Cancer "treatment" in the U.S. has and continues to be a dismal failure. The statistics are terrible. There is considerable question in my mind regarding the advisability of undergoing *any* such so-called "treatments" as chemotherapy, radiation and surgery in most cases, when the success rate is so abysmally low—often *non-*

existent, and the side-effects so severe and destructive. But... that is a subject for another book.

PREVENTIVE MEASURES: The most important of these are intrinsic to the BioSlim program. They are: the avoidance of unnatural, highly processed foods; the avoidance of all added fats and oils, particularly those that are heated; the eating of healthful, life-sustaining, cancer-protective, *real, recognizable* foods such as fresh vegetables, fruits and grains; the ingestion of optimal amounts of *antioxidants,* such as are present in the BioSlim Formulas; and the lifestyle aspects of BioSlim, including the increased activity level, as well as the avoidance of smoking and the searching out of spiritual peace and contentment. The best rule to follow is this: if it's not natural, avoid it. Get out of the pollution, the stress and the junk food; do what nature intended.

It should be noted that the incidence of breast cancer is particularly reducible with a low-added-fat diet such as BioSlim. Other cancers that are most powerfully affected by diet and nutrition (especially fat intake) are: in women, endometrial or cervical (those involving the female uterus and cervix); in men, prostate; and gastrointestinal cancer (stomach, intestinal, liver).

OTHER NUTRITIONAL FACTORS: Many vitamins, minerals and other nutrients are significant in the fight against and prevention of cancer. The most important of these are: vitamin A, folic acid (a B vitamin), vitamin C, vitamin E, bromelain, and the mineral selenium. Each of these is generally available, and is present in optimal dosages in the BioSlim Formulas. There are, in addition, some fascinating new studies going on as this is being written on the effects of a variety of alternative treatments, such as certain herbal remedies, and promisingly, the use of shark liver oil (*alkylglycerols*), of all things. There is not yet sufficient data on these alternative therapies to say definitively that they work, but considering the abysmally poor record of traditional therapy, and the fact that alternative therapies are generally non-toxic and do no harm, they are very well worth keeping an eye on.

♦ CARPAL TUNNEL SYNDROME

This is typified by a syndrome of numbness and pain in the hands, wrists, arms and elbows, usually caused by excessive and/or chronic use or trauma; other possible causes are pregnancy, rheumatoid arthritis, PMS, and other disorders. The pain and numbness is commonly felt in the hand on the side of the palm, and in the first three fingers beginning with the thumb.

Medical treatment consists of rest, ice, and usually, anti-inflammatory medication. Surgery is sometimes necessary.

NUTRITIONAL FACTORS: These are usually very effective in this disorder. The most important factors are: vitamin B6 in doses of 40-100 milligrams per day and the mineral magnesium, in doses of at least 500-1000 milligrams per day. GLA (see ARTHRITIS above) and the bioflavonoids (especially quercetin) may also be helpful.

NOTE: Acupuncture is a great idea, and may well help the sufferer avoid surgery.

♦ CATARACTS

Cataracts are a leading cause of blindness. This condition is defined as *opacification* or clouding of the lens of the eye, which is the structure directly behind the pupil through which all light must pass on its way to the *retina,* the organ that facilitates vision. Cataracts are most commonly "caused" by advancing age, but may be caused or exacerbated by other factors, such as diabetes, certain drugs (steroids, Thorazine, et al), and certain other, often rare disease states (e.g., galactosemia, hypoparathyroidism, Wilson's disease, and certain inflammatory conditions of the eye).

Medical treatment is usually surgical lens replacement.

As always, a tiny sliver of prevention is worth more than all the medical treatment in the world.

NUTRITIONAL FACTORS: Deficiencies of vitamin B2 (riboflavin), vitamin C, vitamin E, and the minerals selenium and zinc have all been implicated in the premature formation of cataracts. Adequate, even higher-than-normal intake of these nutrients is recommended for anyone suffering from or at risk of developing this potentially crippling disorder. Note that all are present in highly appropriate quantities in the BioSlim Formulas.

♦ CHOLESTEROL LEVEL, ELEVATED

Due to massive media attention, nearly every American today worries about his or her cholesterol level.

It has all gone *way* too far.

We are now seeing people with major illnesses—often entirely unrelated to cholesterol levels and cardiovascular disease—whose primary health concern remains focused on cholesterol. The situation has gone beyond reason, and well beyond what the *facts* about cholesterol warrant.

The evidence for a cholesterol–heart disease connection is far ***weaker*** than most people realize and does not in any way justify the level of fear and hyperbole surrounding this issue.

Here are some of the facts:

- Available evidence indicates **no significant correlation between cholesterol levels and heart disease in people who are over approximately 50 years of age**. In women, there is also no significant correlation in anyone who has not yet undergone menopause. Note that the age group where there is no correlation is the very same age group who is at highest risk for heart disease. In other words, **we cannot help those at highest risk of heart disease by worrying about and treating their cholesterol levels!**
- About 75%–85% of all cholesterol in the body is manufactured by the body itself—in every cell, but mostly in the liver; it is, for the most part, NOT obtained from outside sources. It has been shown, for example, that eggs can be eaten in *huge* quantities with negligible effect on cholesterol levels. The body responds to a wide variety of stimuli—

nutritional, biochemical, hormonal and toxic—all of which contribute to the serum cholesterol level we measure.

- Excessive intake of *un*saturated fats, as suggested by most cholesterol-lowering regimens, may lead to an *increase* in the risk for cancer development.
- There are disturbing reports of an *increased* incidence of heart attacks in people taking some of the currently popular cholesterol lowering drugs.
- *Low* cholesterol levels are associated with significantly increased rates of illness and death—a little known fact.
- In many people, dieting alone has little to *no effect* on cholesterol levels. Diet improvement may, however, benefit the health of these same individuals, especially if it is coupled with a good nutritional and exercise program. This can then decrease the overall cardiac risk, which is, after all, the whole point.
- Laboratory cholesterol evaluations are often unreliable due to error and variances caused by individual factors such as time of day, recent food ingestion, blood-drawing method, et al.
- The most common cause of high cholesterol levels in this country is hypothyroidism, a deficiency of the thyroid gland (see THYROID PROBLEMS later in this section for details). This problem cannot be significantly affected by diet alone.
- **Cholesterol levels are essentially statistically relevant ONLY to young and near-middle-aged men under the age of approximately 50.** Even in this group, the correlation is relatively minor.
- Relative values of HDL and LDL ("good" and "bad" cholesterol, respectively) may be far more important overall than actual total cholesterol levels.

* * *

We must *de*-emphasize the importance of cholesterol levels, and instead, focus on the well-known, truly *important* factors affecting the health of the heart and the cardiovascular system, including:

1) The **AVOIDANCE OF SMOKING** — the single greatest contributor to heart disease in America today.

2) A comprehensive and aggressive **NUTRITIONAL PROGRAM** — elimination of obesity and optimal nutrition are key factors, as is the balancing of metabolic states.

3) An **ACTIVITY PROGRAM** — matching each individual's capabilities and cardiovascular health.

4) Comprehensive **MEDICAL HEALTH EVALUATIONS** — to identify those people who are at highest risk. This is important not so that we can bombard more people with drugs, but so that significant, active problems may be recognized and addressed, and so that those people can thereby gain the motivation to begin the kind of health-building program that can truly make a difference. Note that BioSlim is, by design, a *perfect* program for cardiovascular health improvement.

* * *

It is now more important than ever to emphasize a whole-body, comprehensive approach to health. An important point here is that **virtually none of the studies done to date on the possible reduction of heart disease risks through cholesterol level reduction resulted in any significantly increased life-span for the study participants.** It seems that the process used to purportedly *reduce* cardiac risks actually *increased* other health risks, thereby nullifying the overall health "benefit". This may be due, in part, to the negative side-effects of the drugs used in these studies, and to the ill-advised, unbalanced and unnaturally elevated ingestion of unsaturated oils, which may cause other problems in the human body not directly related to the cardiovascular system... such as cancer.

Only by focusing on the _whole_ person, by *minimizing* drug intervention down to that which is truly essential, and by closely following a more responsible, more natural approach to health care, can we positively improve our health.

NUTRITIONAL FACTORS: As above, diet is important, as is a proper activity level. The factors that contribute to high cholesterol levels are, in some sense fortunately, the same as those that cause obesity. This means that by following the BioSlim System you are not only going to lose weight, but can also normalize your blood fat and cholesterol levels. In fact, the BioSlim program is the _perfectly correct_ one for cardiovascular health improvement.

Specific food elements that should be **avoided** include: SATURATED FATS (all fats derived from animal sources, including dairy products), all ADDED FATS (fats processed and added to real food), and REFINED SUGAR. These are actually damaging to your body in many ways, and are best avoided altogether in any event.

Food elements that may be *helpful* include: *fiber*, found in virtually all vegetable, fruits and grains, and *garlic*, found to be directly useful in helping control blood fat and cholesterol levels.

NUTRITIONAL SUPPLEMENTATION: There are many nutrients important to your body's proper handling of cholesterol and fats in general. These include the minerals magnesium, chromium, selenium, manganese and zinc, as well as the vitamins niacin, B6, pantothenic acid, C, E, and folic acid. Also helpful are the Essential Fatty Acids (see the *BioSlim Formulas* chapter, below), and possibly CoQ10. All of the important nutrients are present in correct balance in the BioSlim Formulas; some people may wish to add an Essential Fatty Acid (EFA) supplement. (NOTE: A well-balanced diet, as per the BioSlim Food Plan, should supply plenty of EFAs or EFA precursors.)

♦ COLITIS

The word *"colitis"* has several meanings. It is sometimes used to mean a syndrome of bowel irritation, also called *irritable* bowel syndrome (IBS); more commonly, it refers to a true inflammation of some part of the intestinal tract, also known as *inflammatory bowel disease (IBD)*. Colitis, in its more benign IBS form, can be caused or exacerbated by stress, improper diet, and certain food sensitivities, such as to gluten or milk products. A transient form of colitis can be infectious in origin, as in *infectious gastroenteritis* (commonly called "stomach flu"). The more serious inflammatory kind (IBD) is believed to be caused by a variety of factors: hereditary, environmental, food-related, psychological, auto-immune and allergic.

Symptoms may include abdominal pain/cramping, diarrhea and rectal bleeding. Diagnosis of IBD can be made definitively through a lower GI series (using barium and X-rays), and/or colonoscopy with biopsy, where a long, flexible tube is inserted into the colon and a small biopsy is taken for analysis.

Medical treatment is often difficult, consisting of "bland" diet, inflammation-reducing drugs, and as a last resort, surgical removal of the affected parts of the colon.

PREVENTION: There is evidence linking the ingestion of cow's milk and cow's milk products to colitis. This link is *not* limited to the well-known phenomenon of *lactose intolerance,* which is a very common problem—for some ethnic groups it reaches a prevalence of over 90%—where the sugar in milk, called *lactose,* cannot be properly digested by the body, leading to pain, bloating and diarrhea. While lactose intolerance is very, very common, it does not typically cause a full-blown colitis, though it can be one of the factors predisposing to it. It is, rather, milk itself—i.e., the proteins and other constituents that comprise milk (this includes the milk used in milk products such as cheese, cream, milk powder/concentrate, etc.)—that is the source of the problem. It is best, then, to **avoid all milk and milk products** if you suffer from the symptoms of colitis, even in its mild form.

Cigarette smoking can cause and exacerbate colitis. It must be avoided under all circumstances.

Food sensitivities can exacerbate IBD. The most commonly offending foods include: milk products, gluten-containing cereals (wheat, oat, barley, rye), yeast, corn, nuts, tomatoes (and the other *Nightshades:* potato, eggplant and all peppers; see above under ARTHRITIS), alcohol and chemically treated tap water (always use pure, untreated bottled water). Refined sugar should be avoided. Self-experimentation to root out offending foods is highly recommended, as each individual is unique, and will have his or her own unique set of food sensitivities.

NUTRITIONAL SUPPLEMENTATION: Nutrients that are either found low in patients suffering from colitis, or that may help reduce the severity thereof are: vitamin A, vitamin B_{12}, folic acid, vitamin C, Essential Fatty Acids, and the minerals: magnesium, zinc, iron, selenium and calcium. The BioSlim program may be used by people suffering from colitis with excellent results. Of course, the attention of a personal physician is essential.

One other supplement that may be very helpful is *friendly bowel flora*, which are the normal, beneficial bacteria that usually populate the intestinal tract by the *billions*. These "friendly" bacteria help digest food in the gut, actually synthesize certain vitamins, and in general, keep things moving along healthfully in the digestive tract. They are *essential* to health. Without them, you would soon waste away, and probably die of malnutrition. In colitis and other disease states, as well as after any course of antibiotics, the population of these friendly bacteria may be greatly altered. Replenishing these bacteria can do wonders for the health of anyone suffering from this kind of imbalance.

I routinely recommend such supplementation *whenever* antibiotics are prescribed, and as adjuvant nutritional supplementation in cases of colitis or other gastrointestinal disturbances. These supplements are usually called **lactobacillus** (a general term for the most common form of these friendly bacteria), or *acidophilus* (a form of lactobacillus).

♦ CONSTIPATION

This is a common reaction to any change of diet. It is most often exacerbated by insufficient intake of *water*, which is why it is important to drink plenty (min. 7-8 glasses daily) of pure, chemical-free water, especially if you suffer from constipation.

Other factors that may contribute to constipation include insufficient *fiber* in the diet. Of course, the BioSlim program is intrinsically high in fiber, but it is possible, by concentrating on the animal products (meat, eggs, chicken, fish, milk), to circumvent the intent of the program and end up with a low fiber diet. The best way to avoid this problem is to eat more vegetables (the green kind are best), some fruit, and if eating grains at all, only the *whole* kind. If necessary, a *psyllium* fiber supplement (available in pure form in most health stores and as flavored mix in all pharmacies), can do wonders. If you do take a fiber supplement, **be sure to drink plenty of water with it and throughout the day**, for without sufficient water fiber supplementation can and will make you <u>worse</u>, by congealing in your digestive tract, a bit like concrete would, thereby effectively plugging up your system and worsening your condition.

Lactobacillus (see above under COLITIS) can also help.

Activity level is an important factor in preventing and relieving chronic constipation. Especially helpful are activities that involve the mid-section of the body

The *worst* way to treat constipation is with a laxative, as it accomplishes nothing permanent whatsoever, and can lead to a dependence on its chemical effect. If *necessary*, the one laxative to try is milk of magnesia, since it does not work chemically on the bowel wall, but rather through an *osmotic* effect by increasing the water content of the bowel. And it has the side benefit of providing extra magnesium, an essential mineral, to the body.

For more information on constipation, see the *Solving Problems* section later in this book.

NOTE: There are many nutritional factors important to maintaining proper bowel balance and movement and these are generally incorporated into the BioSlim System. The BioSlim

Formulas are themselves, in fact, designed to gently help keep things moving along.

♦ DIABETES

This is a condition where the hormone *insulin* does not perform its assigned task of regulating the sugar level in the bloodstream, either because of insufficient production by the pancreas or because of its diminished ability to affect the body's cells (*insulin resistance*). Diabetes is a serious disease that afflicts millions of people. It can lead to deterioration of many important organs and systems such as the heart, kidneys, blood vessels, nervous system, eyes, and others. Treatment usually starts first with a controlled diet, then, if necessary, drugs.

There are some facts about this ailment that are not well known, even by many physicians. The first and most important of these is just *how* to adjust the diet to control diabetes, and how *effective* this can be. Most individuals suffering from what is commonly known as "adult onset" diabetes (as opposed to the kind you're born with), can have their condition controlled *without medication,* if the proper diet and nutritional program are followed. Unfortunately, this happens all too infrequently. Too often, the first treatment is oral medication, despite the fact that these medications *increase* the rate of heart disease and *decrease* survival rates due to heart-related illness.

The correct diet for diabetics is one just like BioSlim! Not because it was designed to treat diabetes, but because it is simply the *healthiest* way to eat, and because it just happens to be the case that the same diet and nutritional support that helps people control cravings, lose weight and improve energy levels is also the optimal one for diabetics. In fact, the BioSlim Formulas were originally designed to help maximize the body's ability to control blood sugar levels. This was done in recognition of the fact that cravings are often caused by out-of-control blood sugar levels. People with diabetes, then, can experience the additional benefit of better blood sugar control under the BioSlim System.

Keep in mind: you must be under a physician's care! Especially if you are on any medication. If you begin following the BioSlim program closely, it is possible for your blood sugar to *drop dramatically*—on its own! If you are on medication for diabetes, the drugs you take can cause your body to "overshoot" the mark, which can potentially cause a serious episode of <u>low</u> blood sugar, a condition that is far more immediately dangerous than the chronic high blood sugar most diabetics have.

> CASE HISTORY: A 52 year old man, Arthur, came in complaining of increased thirst and urination. He was worried because his father had died of complications of diabetes, and he had heard that his symptoms could be the hallmarks of the diabetic state. He was right. His fasting blood sugars were elevated to about 400 (normal is up to about 110-120), his urinalysis revealed evidence that his kidneys were starting to suffer from the deterioration commonly caused by diabetes, and there was other laboratory evidence that his diabetes was raging out of control.
>
> I informed Arthur of these facts, and discussed with him what the best approach would be. With a blood sugar this high, I explained, it would be prudent to put him on some form of medication immediately, with a view to reducing or eliminating it when he stabilized. But, I said, if he were highly motivated, we could *try,* for a limited time, to fix his problem without medication, using only diet and nutritional support.
>
> Arthur was game. He was also quite frightened of the disease, as he had seen what it had done to his father. Arthur went on the BioSlim program, and followed it religiously.
>
> Within three days, his symptoms *disappeared.* Approximately four weeks after starting the program, his labs had improved dramatically — the blood sugar and other laboratory parameters were only slightly above normal. After eight weeks, *all* his labs were normal. Currently, his blood sugar indices are on the *low* side! He is on no medication whatsoever, and feels "great".

There are two important lessons to be learned from this case: (1) the body has an amazing ability to heal and right itself—given half a chance. (2) More specifically, it is vital to carefully watch drug dosing in cases of diabetes when a new diet and health-building program is adopted. Had Arthur been taking blood sugar lowering medication when he started his health program, he would soon have found himself in the same position as a normally healthy person taking the same drugs! Since his blood sugars normalized with no medication at all, *with* medication they could easily have become *too low,* posing a potentially serious problem.

If you suffer from diabetes, by all means—start the BioSlim program immediately. But tell your doctor, *especially if you are on any anti-diabetes medication.* In general, it is usually better to start with too little medication and raise it than run the risk of taking too *much* medication for your condition.

♦ FATIGUE, CHRONIC OR SEVERE

Fatigue is a basic symptom that is part of virtually every known illness. It is what is known as a " non-specific" symptom, i.e., it does not point to any specific etiology or cause.

Some of the more common problems that can be confused with a *chronic* fatigue syndrome include:
- chronic disease of any kind,
- chronic inflammation,
- multiple sclerosis,
- cancer,
- most infectious diseases, such as venereal, fungal, bacterial, viral, parasitic, or spirochetal (e.g. Lyme disease or syphilis),
- AIDS,
- hormonal dysfunction (thyroid, adrenal, et al),
- psychological or psychiatric disorders,
- disorders of the blood (such as anemia or a white cell dysfunction),
- lung or heart ailments,
- heavy metal (e.g., lead or mercury) or chemical toxicity,

- multiple environmental allergies and sensitivities,
- auto-immune disorders of all kinds,
- obesity,
- and many others.

Obviously, the list is long, and it could be much longer since fatigue is such a ubiquitous symptom.

There is today, with regard to this symptom, a new entity: *Chronic Fatigue Syndrome* (CFS), defined in part as severe fatigue of substantial duration (typically, at least six months) for which no explanation can be found in the ordinary course of medical evaluation. This is not an easy diagnosis to make, though there are several symptoms and signs that tend to support it, in addition to the underlying severe fatigue, including:

- body and/or joint aches,
- debilitating headaches,
- mild to moderate lymph node swelling,
- muscle weakness,
- confusion and "cognitive dysfunction" (the inability to think clearly and remember well),
- depression and sleep disturbance.
- other "criteria", including several involving blood tests; none is considered definitive for making the diagnosis.

A very aggressive, thorough search for a diagnosis *other* than chronic fatigue syndrome must be undertaken in all suspected cases, because most medical causes of fatigue are treatable, and some are quite serious.

It is important not to fall into the trap of identifying an unexplained syndrome without a complete search for other causes. Keep in mind that the name *Chronic Fatigue Syndrome* is merely a term we use instead of the longer, less attractive, but more accurate description: *"A syndrome of fatigue about which we know almost nothing, and whose cause completely baffles us"*. This latter name is, in fact, what we essentially mean when we label *many* diseases, including this representative list: cancer, chronic fatigue syndrome, lupus, rheumatoid arthritis, thyroiditis, and to a large extent, even heart disease. These are but a few of the many, many diseases that we actually know very little about. The point is: the fact that we are able to name something does not mean that we know much about it, and certainly does not mean that we know how to treat it.

If a specific reason is found for fatigue, it should be treated. This includes all chronic infections, and the somewhat controversial entity of *chronic candidiasis,* a condition of overgrowth of certain fungi in the intestines, vagina, and other body organs (*candida* is a kind of fungus). (See the *Yeast Syndromes* subject in the *Women: Special Facts and Considerations* chapter below for more on this subject.)

Keep in mind that the diagnosis of *Chronic Fatigue Syndrome* has been expanded, so that the current full name is *Chronic Fatigue And Immune Deficiency Syndrome* (CFIDS), because along with chronic, severe fatigue, many sufferers also manifest diminished immune system capabilities.

If the diagnosis of *Chronic Fatigue Syndrome* is made, an aggressive program of nutritional and psychological support should be instituted. The best approach to the nutritional aspects of a program to combat fatigue is, luckily, the one embodied in the BioSlim System.

NUTRITIONAL FACTORS: Diet should be as pure and clear of processed, adulterated food as possible. Obesity should be eliminated. Avoid sugar in all its forms, as well as all added fats and all milk products. Avoid all foods to which you may be allergic or in any way sensitive.

Both the BioSlim Formulas should be taken in full doses. Additional magnesium (for a total of 800 to 1000 milligrams per day) and calcium (also a total of 800 to 1000 milligrams per day) should be taken. Other important specific nutrients, all present in full doses in the BioSlim Formulas, include: vitamin B6, pantothenic acid (a B vitamin), vitamin B12, vitamin C, iron, and zinc.

SPECIAL ADDITIONAL NUTRITIONAL FACTORS: The amino acid (protein building block) *aspartic acid* can be very helpful, especially in the form of *magnesium-potassium aspartate* (800–1000 mg per day). Coenzyme Q10 (CoQ10), Essential Fatty Acids, and *lactobacillus* (friendly intestinal bacteria), have also been found helpful.

♦ GALLSTONES

Gallstones are usually composed of cholesterol and/or calcium. They form in the area of the liver and gallbladder, and can cause severe abdominal pain, mostly in the upper right side of the abdomen, particularly after fat-containing meals. More severe consequences include blockage of the flow of material (bile) from the liver to the intestines and full-blown inflammation of the gallbladder ("cholecystitis") or bile ducts ("cholangitis"). The best way to prevent these is to prevent the formation of gallstones.

NUTRITIONAL FACTORS: The best nutritional program to help minimize gallstone formation is a diet low in all fats, moderate in calories, and high in fiber. Avoidance of obesity is a major factor. Nutritional supplementation that may be helpful includes: vitamin A, the B-vitamins, vitamin C and vitamin E (all present in balanced form in the BioSlim Formulas). Additional Essential Fatty Acids may also be helpful, as may fiber supplements such as psyllium seed husk powder.

In general, a diet high in vegetables, and some fruit, combined with appropriate attention to nutrition is the key. The BioSlim plan fits this description well, and should well reward those with a propensity for the development of gallstones.

♦ HAY FEVER

See ALLERGIES above.

♦ HEADACHES

This is one of the most common complaints in the world. Some people, suffer from severe, recurrent headaches called *migraines,* that can be quite debilitating. These severely painful headaches come in various forms, called *classic* or *common,* or *cluster.* Migraines belong to the *vascular* type of headache.

There are essentially three general kinds of headaches: *tension* headaches, resulting from muscle tension or spasm in the neck, scalp or forehead; *sinus* headaches, resulting from inflammation of the membranes lining the nasal sinuses; and *vascular* headaches, stemming from spasm or other dysfunction in the vessels inside the head, in and around the brain.

Some possible causes of headaches are: trauma anywhere in the head or neck, diseases of the eyes, ears, nose or throat, certain drugs, alcohol, cigarette smoke, air pollution, food sensitivities or allergies, any allergy, anemia, hypoglycemia (low blood sugar), excessive salt intake, menopause, birth control pills, PMS (pre-menstrual syndrome, dental disease, the grinding of teeth during night or day ("*bruxism*"), TMJ syndrome (a painful condition of the area just in front of the ear where the jaw meets the face), fever from any source, and any chronic illness.

Medical treatment usually consists of removing any known causative factors or diseases, and drugs. Drugs, unfortunately, usually do nothing about the underlying problem, merely masking the pain. New drugs, such as *sumatryptan* (aka: *Imitrex*), can be very effective, particularly in certain cases of migraine headache.

Of course, such common headache-causing diseases as sinusitis and neck muscle spasm should be dealt with first when treating headaches.

Acupuncture is often a very helpful treatment modality, and is highly recommended, as is relaxation therapy and biofeedback.

NUTRITIONAL FACTORS: Caffeine has an interesting relationship to headaches: It can both cause the vascular kinds and alleviate them. If you are one of the many people who drink coffee every day, be aware that you are probably addicted to it by now.

We define "addicted" here as physically dependent, which is what you may well be. How can you tell? Try stopping the coffee "cold turkey". If you're like most heavy coffee drinkers, you'll probably have a headache every day for 5–7 days after stopping caffeine. This is a *withdrawal response*: it means you are physically "dependent" on caffeine. Note: *caffeine is a drug!*

Coffee can be a direct cause of vascular headaches. If you suffer from headaches and drink coffee, you should stop. The best way to break a coffee addiction is to gradually taper down your caffeine ingestion over a period of approximately two weeks. This should minimize withdrawal symptoms. Also, be sure to include in your diet some high quality nutritional support.

Avoiding food sensitivities is often important to the prevention of headaches, though difficult to do. The best approach is personal experimentation, during which keeping a careful record of all ingested foods and resultant symptoms is vital. The avoidance of all milk products and all forms of sugar is highly recommended.

It is interesting to note how often headaches are associated with gastrointestinal problems, especially constipation, which should be treated aggressively in such cases. See the CONSTIPATION section above for treatments thereof.

SPECIFIC NUTRIENTS that may be helpful include: vitamin B6 (particularly for women with hormone-related headaches), magnesium, zinc (particularly for cluster headaches), niacin and calcium. All are in the BioSlim Formulas. The Essential Fatty Acids and the two natural herbs, *Feverfew* and *Angelica sinensis* (aka: Dong Quai or Tang Kwei) may also be helpful.

As you get healthier and improve overall, your headaches should diminish and finally disappear, assuming you are given a clean bill of health by your physician. And don't forget your Activity Plan, which can also help relieve chronic headaches.

♦ HEART DISEASE / CARDIOVASCULAR DISORDERS

> NOTE: Anyone with a serious disorder of the heart should begin this and *any* program of activity and nutritional support *slowly* and *carefully*. This means that any exercise or increased activity program and the doses of the Formulas should be started at low levels, then increased gradually, as tolerated. The supervision of a physician is essential.

The heart is at once the strongest, most durable muscle of the body, and the most sensitive. It pumps life-sustaining blood throughout the circulatory system, including vessels that in turn feed the muscle of the heart itself. These tiny blood vessels are called the *"coronary arteries"* in recognition of the crown-like structure they form on the surface of the heart.

When the blood vessels of the body become congested and clogged, the vessels that are most susceptible are those feeding the heart (the coronary arteries) and the ones feeding the brain. A complete blockage of a coronary artery causes a *heart attack*, while vessel blockage in the brain causes a *stroke*. In either case, the underlying mechanism of the problem is similar: for one reason or another, the blood vessel is no longer able to carry blood to the organ involved, which causes parts of that organ to die — i.e., a heart attack or a stroke occurs.

Arteries can be *partially* blocked, causing insufficient blood supply. This causes chest pain or *angina* in the heart, and mini-strokes known as *TIAs* ("Transient Ischemic Attacks") in the brain. These transient insufficiencies of blood supply are much more common than full-blown blockages, one reason for which is that full blockages can only happen a very few times before death occurs, while it is possible for insufficiencies to occur hundreds of times in one individual. If an artery feeding the heart is partially blocked, chest pain may occur under any conditions that cause blood to flow more heavily to other parts of the body, thereby placing a strain on the heart and causing it to require more blood to function properly. This extraordinary requirement for blood by the heart itself cannot then be easily supplied because of the partial blockage(s) that exist(s) in the coronary arteries feeding it. Activities that can precipitate chest pain under these conditions include: large meals, exertion of any kind, stress of any kind, and exposure to cold.

Of course, any heart condition must be treated by a physician. Medical treatment usually consists of drugs and/or surgery. Diet and lifestyle are usually addressed via the admonitions to eat less fat and stop smoking.

There has been a tremendous amount of research done in recent decades on the causes of heart disease and *atherosclerosis,* the process by which arteries become clogged. Much has been written on the effects of elevated cholesterol levels, though for the most part, this concept is far less relevant than most people believe. (See CHOLESTEROL LEVEL, ELEVATED above.)

For many years, we were told to eat more unsaturated oils. Now, with the possible exception of olive oil, this advice has been found to be baseless, even potentially harmful. Eating more unsaturated oil does nothing to prevent heart disease, and may well increase the risk of certain other diseases, especially cancer, and may even *increase* the risk of heart disease itself!

PREVENTION: Stopping the smoking of cigarettes is the single most effective measure any smoker can take to prevent heart disease. Weight reduction in cases of obesity is important. Controlling blood pressure is important; it may be accomplished through dietary measures as well as relaxation methods. Of course, out-of-control blood pressure must be treated by a physician. Reasonable physical activity is also an important preventive measure.

Essentially, the BioSlim program can be thought of as good therapy for the heart, since it is perfectly suited for that task, and intrinsically contains the necessary elements listed here.

NUTRITIONAL FACTORS: **The importance of avoiding added fats cannot be overemphasized**. Just as this rule is the primary principle of the BioSlim program, so too is it the most important dietary measure you can take to help prevent and, in fact, *reverse* heart disease. This is true for many reasons, including the general importance of fat reduction and, less commonly known, the fact that certain kinds of fat molecules—the *trans* fatty acids caused by the *processing* and *heating* of unsaturated fat—appear to be directly responsible for atherosclerosis, the plugging up of blood vessels in the body.

A diet high in fiber is also very helpful.

NUTRITIONAL SUPPLEMENTATION includes most of the vitamins and minerals, such as: vitamin A, vitamin B6, folic acid, niacin, vitamin C, vitamin E, **magnesium**, chromium, selenium, iodine, zinc, and others. All are present in correct balance in the BioSlim Formulas.

Additional potentially helpful supplementation includes the Essential Fatty Acids (EFAs), bromelain, CoQ10, extract of the plant ginkgo bilboa, and garlic. CoQ10 and magnesium have also been found helpful in certain heart arrhythmias (irregular heart beats).

People with such relatively common disorders as irregular or fast heart beats (*arrhythmias* and *tachycardias*) and *mitral valve prolapse* can use the BioSlim System and may well find that their symptoms improve on the program.

Historically, heart disease is a fairly new disease, partly because people are living longer, but mostly because of the preponderance of *non-foods* being consumed today in place of real, whole, natural, *recognizable* food. This is an area where you can do much to prevent disease and premature death. The BioSlim System is one way to accomplish just that, while in the bargain, dropping as much weight as you need to lose.

♦ HEMORRHOIDS

Hemorrhoids are caused by the pressure of blood in the *hemorrhoidal veins*, a collection of blood vessels in the area of the anus. The word *hemorrhoids* is commonly defined as a swelling of those veins. This swelling can lead to bleeding from the affected veins, or pain, or both.

The most common cause of hemorrhoids is constipation, since the pressure of straining at stool causes tremendous backup pressure in the veins of the anus. Therefore, avoidance of constipation, and of all activities that increase pressure inside the abdomen or on the hemorrhoidal veins should be avoided. (Sit-ups, lifting heavy weights and running, for example, are not good ideas. Swimming and stair climbing are.)

The medical treatment here consists of the avoidance of constipation, sitz baths, and in severe cases, surgery.

Exercise can be very helpful, but as noted, not the kind that increases pressure in the abdomen or on the hemorrhoidal veins. Clothing that is tight around the waist or pelvic areas should be avoided, as should prolonged sitting.

NUTRITIONAL FACTORS: Lots of water throughout the day, in conjunction with a high fiber diet is very helpful. Psyllium seed husks can be helpful as a fiber supplement, with plenty of water. Avoid dairy foods, and most other animal products. Bioflavonoids may help, through their function in helping to strengthen blood vessel walls. Vitamin B6, vitamin C, vitamin E, and magnesium are also recommended.

The BioSlim System is an excellent one for sufferers of this ailment, as it emphasizes the right balance of foods and is nutritionally correct. Note that the BioSlim Formulas were designed to help keep things moving properly in the bowels, and would therefore be helpful in the prevention of hemorrhoids.

♦ HIGH BLOOD PRESSURE (HYPERTENSION)

Blood pressure is the pressure with which blood is being forced through the body's blood vessels. Blood pressure rises and falls all the time. For example, exercising naturally causes blood pressure to rise temporarily. This is the way the body is able to get more blood to the parts of the body that need it. It is perfectly normal. Sometimes, though, blood pressure *stays* elevated, and it is then that it can become dangerous.

High blood pressure is a very common problem. It is a disease with very few symptoms until it reaches life-threatening levels. For this reason, it is often called "the silent killer". Usually, the only way to diagnose it is by having your blood pressure checked. By the time actual symptoms, such as headaches, nosebleeds, or blurred vision occur, it is likely that an advanced stage of this disease has been reached. The time to treat is *before* it reaches this level.

The most common form of hypertension has no known organic cause and is called "essential hypertension".

Note that hypertension can also be caused by dysfunction in such organs as the kidneys, heart, blood vessels, and adrenals.

Medical treatment usually consists of salt restriction, stress reduction and most commonly, drugs.

The preventive and nutritional factors that can affect this disease are very similar to those listed above under HEART DISEASE / CARDIOVASCULAR DISORDERS and CHOLESTEROL LEVELS, ELEVATED. It should be noted that recent work in the field indicates that it is not so much the avoidance of sodium (as in table salt) that is important, as the proper ingestion of sufficient amounts of *potassium*. Potassium is a mineral that acts in tandem with—in a sense, at cross purposes to—sodium in the body. It is found in large quantities in foods of plant origin (vegetables, fruits, whole grains).

Garlic and *taurine* (an amino acid) may also be helpful.

Stress reduction is an important tool in controlling blood pressure. One of the best ways to accomplish this is with a technique called *biofeedback,* which is highly recommended.

Regular aerobic activity is also very important in the treatment and prevention of this disease.

♦ KIDNEY STONES

This is an extremely painful disorder of stone formation in the highly sensitive area of the kidneys and its associated plumbing. These stones are most commonly made of calcium and a substance called *oxalate,* found in such foods as spinach, rhubarb, dandelion greens, chocolate or cocoa, cashews, almonds, and (non-herbal) tea. All these foods should be avoided by anyone suffering from kidney stones, unless the stones are known to be other than the oxalate-containing variety, such as *uric acid* stones (sometimes present with gout).

Medical treatment consists of aggressive fluid administration, drugs for pain relief, and in severe cases, surgery.

NUTRITIONAL FACTORS: These can be very effective in eliminating this problem, thus perhaps avoiding surgery. The most important factors are **magnesium** and **vitamin B6**. Aggressive supplementation with these two nutrients alone can have a remarkably beneficial effect on this disease. Both are in the BioSlim Formulas.

Other potentially helpful nutrients include: protein (adequate, but not overly high amounts), vitamin A, vitamin B2 and vitamin C. Individuals with *uric acid* or *cystine* stones (only) should *limit* their protein intake and eat plenty of fruits and vegetables to keep the urine alkaline (non-acidic).

All persons with kidney stones should drink copious amounts of fluids throughout each day, avoiding dehydration at all costs.

♦ LUNG DISORDERS

This category includes many diverse ailments. The most common are *infectious* (upper respiratory infection, bronchitis, pneumonia) and *obstructive* (asthma, chronic obstructive pulmonary disease or COPD).

Some individuals are particularly prone to respiratory ailments. They may come down with some kind of lung illness several times per year, often punctuated by bouts of pneumonia. Such persons can often be greatly helped by a *preventive* approach to their problem, as opposed to treatment limited to the administration of antibiotics for each acute episode.

ASTHMA is a common disease that can be ultimately life-threatening. It is a condition where the tubes that carry air in the lungs (*bronchi*) contract abnormally and excessively, thereby blocking the normal flow of air into the lungs and causing the characteristic *wheezing* sound that is the hallmark of the disease. The reasons for this abnormal contraction are not fully known, but it is often caused by an allergic reaction to something in the air. Anything can trigger a reaction. Severe, life-threatening asthmatic reactions are known to occur after eating certain foods, such as the *nitrites* used in foods like certain processed forms of meat and some wines.

The medical treatment of lung-related diseases usually consists of antibiotics for infections and allergen avoidance and "lung expanding" drugs for asthma.

PREVENTIVE MEASURES: For people suffering from chronic lung infections, this must include the complete cessation of smoking. Smoking directly and continuously irritates the lining of the lungs, and will cause repeated bouts of infections in susceptible individuals.

Other steps include the avoidance of air pollutants, adequate fluid intake and regular deep breathing. Deep breathing is something that few people do consciously. An occasional sigh is the only opportunity most individuals have to take a deep breath. So it is important to remember to do this consciously and regularly, especially if you are not exercising regularly.

Regular physical activity can be very beneficial to sufferers chronic lung infections.

Avoidance of food allergens, particularly all milk and milk products, is especially helpful.

Nutritional supplementation for persons with chronic lung infections: vitamin A (a total of 25,000 I.U. per day with food as an initial 1-to-2-week-maximum dose, after which what is in your multivitamin should suffice), vitamin C, zinc. *N-acetyl-cysteine* may also be helpful. *Echinacea* is useful for acute infections. Note: the nutrients listed here are all balanced in the BioSlim Formulas.

FOR ASTHMATICS, once again, the most important preventive element is the avoidance of smoke.

In addition, asthmatics must avoid cold air, which can trigger an immediate relapse. Avoidance of air pollution is also important, as is the removal of all known allergens (allergy-causing substances). Beds should be changed frequently, on the order of twice weekly, to avoid accumulation of microscopic creatures called *mites* that can trigger an asthma attack. Air filters, particularly the kind known as HEPA, can be very helpful, especially in the bedroom at night. A dry environment in the home is important to prevent the accumulation of molds.

NUTRITIONAL SUPPLEMENTATION FOR PERSONS WITH ASTHMA: Vitamin A, pantothenic acid (a B vitamin), vitamin B6, vitamin B_{12}, selenium, and especially **magnesium** may all be helpful. All these nutrients are generally available, and all are present in correct balance in the BioSlim Formulas. The herb *ephedra* is also helpful in many cases, but should be used with caution and under the care of a health professional familiar with its properties (see *Nutrition* chapter above for more on ephedra).

Remember: asthmatics can be allergic to anything; be careful anytime you add anything new to your environment or diet.

♦ MULTIPLE SCLEROSIS (MS)

This is a chronic disease affecting the linings of nerves whose cause is not fully understood. Symptoms include episodes of neurological problems such as visual disturbances, dizziness, muscle weakness (especially in the face) speech difficulties, and disturbances in the ability to properly move the arms and/or legs. These episodes typically wax and wane over time, and may disappear altogether for as long as 20 or 30 years before recurring.

All persons with MS should be under the care of a physician. Medical treatment, though, is strictly supportive. There is no known cure.

Nutritional factors in this disease are indeed vital. Properly following all recommendations can lead to significant improvement, according to several studies done around the world.

NUTRITIONAL FACTORS: The diet should include high levels of cold-processed unsaturated oils. This is a departure from the general BioSlim recommendation of no added oils, and is an exception due to unusual circumstance. Other dietary elements include large amounts of vegetables, fruits and whole grains. Smoking and alcohol must be avoided.

Aggressive supplementation with the B-vitamins (including vitamin B_{12}), cold-processed unsaturated oils, vitamin E, lecithin (usually as a soybean-derived extract), magnesium and zinc may all be helpful, in addition to a complete nutritional program. The BioSlim System may be used as a good basis for this program, with the addition of the oils, lecithin and extra vitamin E.

♦ OSTEOPOROSIS

This is defined as a reduction of the total bone mass of the body, which causes the bones to be "brittle". Its prevalence rises with age. Older women are particularly susceptible to this disease, as it is thought that after menopause, the hormone *estrogen* is no longer available in sufficient quantities to keep the bones of the body strong, as it does in younger women.

For years, it was thought that the aggressive treatment of thyroid deficiencies could cause an exacerbation of osteoporosis. Recent findings indicate that this is not the case.

Many women are placed on estrogen replacement therapy to prevent osteoporosis. My own view is that if estrogen is needed for other reasons, it may be used. But osteoporosis is best prevented and treated using appropriate dietary factors and physical activity. If nature had intended women to take estrogen after menopause, all women would have little pill dispensers built into their bodies. As often happens in these modern times, the "science" of medicine often steps over the boundary of wisdom into the area of arrogance. The fact is that estrogen is one of the primary stimulants of the most common forms of breast cancer, and also abnormally stimulates the lining of the uterus when taken by post-menopausal women—in whom nature intended estrogen levels to remain very low. There is good reason to believe that there is an increased probability of breast and uterine cancer occurring in women taking long-term estrogen after menopause.

Some will say: "There is no perfect evidence that this is the case". But in fact, it is far wiser to say: "There is no evidence that this is *not* true, and plenty of suspicion. Therefore, let us be cautious and humble in the face of the natural order of things, until such time as we can prove beyond a doubt that there is no risk in doing this thing".

PREVENTIVE FACTORS: The most important of these are (a) nutritional and (b) physical activity.

Nutritional factors include the avoidance of sugar and other processed foods, appropriate nutritional intake by about the age of 30, and adequate amounts of calcium, magnesium, manganese, copper, vitamin C, vitamin D and a moderate amount of protein (non-animal sources are best). The avoidance of smoking cannot be overemphasized. A diet low in salt is preferred.

A complete, balanced nutritional program is important. BioSlim is perfectly suited for anyone suffering from or worried about osteoporosis. In addition to the BioSlim Formulas, extra calcium and magnesium should be taken, so that the total daily intake is at least 1000 milligrams of calcium and at least 750 milligrams of magnesium. Most supplements work well, but the best of calcium are made with *micro-crystalline hydroxyapatite.*

♦ PREGNANCY

Of course, pregnancy is not a disease, though at times it may be treated as such by some in the medical profession.

Certain nutrients are required by the pregnant woman in larger-than-normal amounts, such as folic acid, calcium and iron. Alcohol, smoking and practically all drugs should be avoided.

There are many brands of specifically formulated PRE-NATAL nutritional supplements available today. Most of them are of good quality, though the ones available at your local health store are generally better than the ones in your pharmacy.

Though there is no evidence or known reason to not use the BioSlim Formulas, we nevertheless recommend that pregnant women NOT use them, but instead use specific PRENATAL products. This advice will hold until such time as BioSlim formulates a specific pre-natal product. Though the Vita/Min Plus product *could* be used with additional supplementation, it is not recommended.

As soon as pregnancy is over, the BioSlim Formulas may again be used; they are entirely safe and OK with breast feeding.

♦ PROSTATE ENLARGEMENT

This condition occurs in almost 90% of all men, if they get to be old enough. It causes an inability to fully empty the urinary bladder as well as loss of bladder control. Medical treatment usually consists of surgery. Recently a new drug, *finasteride*, has become available and is being touted by its manufacturer as effective in reducing prostate enlargement. Studies have shown a slight reducing effect, with an approximately 5% rate of impotence as the primary side effect identified to date. (See below for a safer, more natural alternative.)

Note: the prostate should be examined regularly by a qualified physician to search for the possibility of prostate cancer.

NUTRITIONAL FACTORS: Prostate enlargement responds well to a nutritional approach. Zinc is a vital nutrient. A well balanced diet with attention to good nutrition is helpful. The BioSlim program is an excellent choice for people with this ailment.

The most effective non-drug, nutritional supplement in use for many years is the extract of the plant *seronoa repens,* also known as *saw palmetto.* Results in several studies using this natural extract have been considerably *better* than those using drug therapy, and with no known side effects. A *standardized extract* is the best form of this nutritional supplement.

♦ SKIN WRINKLING

This condition is included here because many people who lose weight find their skin sagging and wrinkling. This is to be expected whenever there is a significant general loss of body fat because when the layer of fat under the skin (the *subcutaneous fat*) is diminished, the skin will no longer be "puffed out", and may sag. The best way to avoid this is to: (a) not lose weight too quickly, giving the skin a chance to assume its new dimensions properly; (b) avoid exposure to sun; and (c) use a good, all-natural skin moisturizing cream every day (the best example of which is the ***Biotique*™** Day/Night Moisturizer by Medicus). Treat your skin gently, avoiding at all costs excessive drying and the use of chemicals.

♦ STRESS

Stress can be emotional or physical. Either way, it is defined here as the kind that hinders and disturbs. (Note that some stress can be beneficial, as is the stress of strenuous exercise.) Anxiety is the natural companion of stress.

Relaxation therapy can do wonders in many cases. So can *biofeedback*, a system whereby you can learn how to control your thoughts and reactions.

Perhaps the most effective stress reliever of all is the thought best expressed by Abraham Lincoln, a man who suffered greatly through most of his adult life, knowing a kind of stress that most of us cannot imagine. He once remarked: "It is said an Eastern monarch once charged his wise men to invent him a sentence to be ever in view, and which should be true and appropriate in all times and situations. They presented him the words: 'And this, too, shall pass away.' How much it expresses! How chastening in the hour of pride! How consoling in the depths of affliction!"

Ol' Abe had a good point there. Much of what is so troublesome to us today is often gone tomorrow. So why let today's concerns worry us so? Tomorrow, things usually improve. Especially now that you've begun this program. Your appearance and health are sure to benefit greatly. And with this inevitable improvement should come either the solutions to most of your problems or the realization that they were not all so terrible in the first place.

PREVENTIVE AND NUTRITIONAL FACTORS: These include many of the nutrients found in the BioSlim Formulas, especially the B-vitamins, vitamin C, magnesium and calcium. Physical activity or exercise can do wonders for relieving and preventing stress. A good massage, a hot bath, and acupuncture are all modalities that can help, at times enormously. Finally, yoga is one way by which many people find peace and emotional tranquillity.

♦ THYROID GLAND DISEASE

The thyroid gland is in many ways a *master* gland. Directly or indirectly, it controls the functions of most of the body's systems and organs. The thyroid is like the body's gas pedal. It controls how fast your engine runs, how much fuel it burns, how quickly your heart beats, how your digestive system works, how well your immune system functions, even how well your brain works. It is the master controller of your metabolic rate, and as such, is vital to your success in the BioSlim program.

Thyroid hormone deficiency or *hypothyroidism* is a very common, quite troubling disorder that often causes a multitude of confusing symptoms. This is the thyroid disorder on which we shall focus most here. In addition to hypothyroidism, the other most common non-cancerous diseases of the thyroid are *hyper*-thyroidism (excessively high levels of thyroid hormone) and *thyroiditis* (inflammation of the thyroid). All these disorders should be treated by a physician.

*Hyper*thyroidism causes the opposite of *hypo*thyroidism: the body is in high gear, racing all the time. Thyroiditis is a disorder, often auto-immune in nature, where the thyroid becomes inflamed, thereby at times releasing too much thyroid hormone into the bloodstream, and at most other times too little as it is depleted of stored hormone and unable to manufacture more. Thyroiditis should be suspected whenever there is unexplained heart rhythm disturbances, diarrhea, anxiety, insomnia and weight loss, particularly in the first year or so after pregnancy, which is when thyroiditis is most likely to strike. It is often treated by giving thyroid hormone orally, thereby suppressing the body's own thyroid gland activity, allowing a period of dormancy and healing.

HYPOTHYROIDISM is most often found in women. And its incidence increases with age. Therefore, older women have a quite high probability of developing this disorder. (Note that the incidence is not small in women of all ages.)

Symptoms and signs include: fatigue, weight gain, sensitivity to cold or "cold extremities", constipation, dry skin and/or hair, depression, insomnia or hypersomnia (excessive sleepiness), diminished sex drive, irregular menstruation, heavy menstrual flow with excessive cramping, anemia, confusion and cognitive dysfunction (inability to think and/or remember clearly).

Diagnosis is usually done through lab blood tests. Unfortunately, contrary to commonly held opinion (including those of many doctors), blood tests are *not* always definitive. It is possible to have a "normal" set of lab results and be *clinically* hypothyroid. The underarm *basal body temperature test,* where one's temperature is taken immediately upon awakening before anything else is done, may be useful in helping to confirm suspicion; but it too is not perfectly reliable, and certainly not definitive. (This *basal* {"underlying"} temperature may be taken on any day by men and post-menopausal women, and by menstruating women on the second and third days after flow begins. Hypothyroidism may be suspected if the temperature on awakening is *consistently* below 97.8°F.)

The blood tests most important to the diagnosis of hypothyroidism are the HIGHLY SENSITIVE TSH (*Thyroid Stimulating*

Hormone) and the FREE T4 or T7 tests. The TSH test measures how much effort the *pituitary* gland, which controls the thyroid gland, is putting out to try to get the thyroid to work properly. Since TSH is used by the pituitary gland to get the thyroid to work harder, the higher the level of TSH, the more powerful this pituitary effort is. The action of the pituitary gland is used as a good marker for the *weakness* of the thyroid gland. The harder the pituitary works, which means the higher the TSH, the weaker the thyroid gland function may be concluded to be. It's as if the pituitary is "beating a dead horse". TSH levels can sometimes reach levels 30 or more times normal, as the pituitary keeps trying ever harder to get the "dead" thyroid gland to respond.

The FREE T4 or T7 tests directly measure the level of hormone activity in the blood. They are considered *less* accurate than the TSH test. Always insist on a TSH test if hypothyroidism is suspected. Though it should be, it is *not* always done, particularly if you are seeing a general practitioner as opposed to a hormone specialist (endocrinologist) or knowledgeable internist.

If all tests are normal, then strict attention to symptoms must be paid, and a *therapeutic trial* considered. A therapeutic trial is the giving of thyroid hormone to an individual suspected of hypothyroidism, with all effects observed over a period of approximately one month. A positive change in symptoms is taken to mean that the extra hormone is needed, while no change means further testing and investigation may be needed.

Medical treatment of hypothyroidism is via replacement of the missing thyroid hormone using an oral preparation (pill). There are two broad kinds of thyroid hormone drugs available: synthetic (e.g., *Synthroid*) and natural bovine extracts (e.g., *Armour Thyroid*). Most endocrinologists prefer the synthetic kind. Others, I among them, prefer the natural extract, mostly because its contents more closely resemble the hormones produced by the human thyroid in its natural state.

INTERACTION WITH BIOSLIM: **If you have this disorder, it is vital that the diagnosis be made and correct treatment begun**

if the BioSlim program is going to help you succeed to your fullest potential. Hypothyroidism is very common and easy to miss. If you are hypothyroid, without treatment you will probably *never* reach your goals, often without knowing why. Its like banging on a closed door—hopeless. The treatment of hypothyroidism is simple, highly effective, and non-toxic. It must be done properly.

NUTRITIONAL FACTORS: The mineral iodine must be taken in sufficient quantities. Essential Fatty Acids may also be helpful, as they are the building blocks from which thyroid hormone is manufactured by the body.

Complete nutritional support is essential in hypothyroidism, as most of the body's functions are usually depressed and in need of help. The BioSlim System is quite proper for sufferers of hypothyroidism, and may be expected to help all around.

♦ ULCERS (STOMACH AND DUODENAL)

Ulcers are deteriorations—holes—in the lining of the stomach or upper small intestines (a region known as the "duodenum"). This disease is known to be exacerbated by excess stomach acidity, but may occur in cases of normal acidity as well. It is often associated with infection by an organism called *Helicobacter*.

The early stage of eventual ulcer disease is often *gastritis,* which literally means "inflammation of the stomach".

Symptoms may include abdominal pain, "heartburn", and sometimes, back pain. If the ulcer is severe and bleeding occurs, vomiting, diarrhea, black stools, anemia, dizziness and all other symptoms associated with internal bleeding may occur.

Ulcers are a life-threatening disorder. In 20%-30% of all cases, the only symptom or sign is internal bleeding, which can be extremely serious. All ulcers must be treated by a physician, and all symptoms that suggest ulcers must always be taken very seriously.

Medical treatment of ulcer disease consists of acid reducing medications, dietary changes, antibiotics and medications for improving healing or protecting the involved areas. Surgery may be necessary in severe cases.

There are some known causes of this disease, including: **smoking, alcohol, coffee, tea, spicy foods, and** *stress*. Some include **milk products** in this list.

Stress is a major factor and should be minimized as much as possible. Remember: "stress" is entirely determined by the mind of the person experiencing it. The same circumstances that are *"stressful"* to one person may be deemed *"challenging"* by another. We make our own stress. We can *un*make it. Biofeedback and direct stress reduction therapy are two modalities by which this issue can be successfully addressed.

PREVENTIVE AND NUTRITIONAL FACTORS: Avoiding the causative influences mentioned above is vital. Also avoid over-the-counter calcium-based antacids, as they often cause a "rebound" phenomenon whereby *more* acid is produced by the stomach than would otherwise be made there. In other words, they may significantly *worsen* the problem.

A diet high in fiber is helpful. Sugar should be avoided, as should the other offending items listed above. In general, smaller, more frequent meals are preferred to larger, less frequent ones. Sleeping on 2-3 pillows can help avoid reflux of food from the stomach into the esophagus ("food pipe") and the resultant *esophagitis* that can cause.

Nutrients that may help: vitamin A, vitamin B6, vitamin C (taken with food), vitamin E, zinc and the bioflavonoids. (All these are balanced in the BioSlim Formulas.) Additional supplementation may include *lactobacillus*, or friendly, beneficial intestinal bacteria, available in capsule or liquid form. A comprehensive nutritional program is very important.

Of particular interest are: *aloe vera* extract, taken internally as a drink, and *cabbage* extract (sometimes called vitamin U). Comfrey tea has traditionally been widely used, but has recently been suspected of causing harm to the liver.

The BioSlim program is perfectly suitable for, and can be directly beneficial to, persons suffering from ulcer disease.

♦ VAGINITIS / YEAST INFECTIONS

This is a common ailment affecting millions of women each year. It is an inflammation of the lining of the vagina usually caused by infection by yeast (fungus) or bacteria. In older women, it may occur without infection due to the natural thinning of the vaginal lining that occurs with menopause (*atrophic vaginitis*)

The most common organism that causes this vexing problem is the fungus *candida*. This infection can be transmitted sexually, but may also arise internally from the normally present candida in the intestinal tract. (For more information, see *Yeast Syndromes* in the *Women: Special Facts and Considerations* chapter below.)

Symptoms are obvious to anyone who has ever suffered from this disorder: itching or burning, and white, cheesy, malodorous discharge heralds the fungal infection. Other kinds of discharge indicate other infections.

Medical treatment usually consists of anti-fungal medication applied to/in the area, and sometimes taken orally.

PREVENTIVE MEASURES: Good hygiene is very important. Loose, cotton underwear is highly recommended, as is the avoidance of any hosiery or clothing that blocks normal air circulation. Simultaneous treatment of sexual partners is highly recommended to avoid passing the infection back and forth during and/or after treatment. Sugar should be avoided in all its forms, as should junk food, particularly products containing processed, white flour.

NUTRITION:: This must include a *lactobacillus* or *acidophilus* supplement. These friendly bacteria tend to displace fungal elements and other "unfriendly" organisms in the intestinal tract and vagina. Douching with lactobacillus may also be helpful, as can taking garlic, grapefruit seed extract, or caprylic acid.

A well-rounded nutritional program, such as BioSlim, is important.

* * *

NOTE: Any medical condition should be treated by a physician—especially if you are planning on increasing your activity level, reducing your calorie intake level, or in any way significantly changing your diet.

ELEVEN

NEVER "GO ON A DIET" AGAIN!

Dieting is useless. Worse than useless — it can be directly harmful to your health. To illuminate this vital concept, here is a review of important information about dieting and weight regulation:

- Fully ninety-five percent (95%), or 19 out of 20 people who go on diets fail to reach their goals. Of the remaining 5%, approximately 80% (4 out of the 5%) will *regain* the weight they lost, as do most of the original 95% who may lose weight (temporarily) but never reach their goals. **Weight loss achieved through most forms of temporary calorie restriction (i.e., "dieting") is virtually always doomed to failure.** The human body responds to intermittent calorie restriction by learning to live with less calories—by *reducing the metabolic rate* of the dieter. Combined with the lean-body-weight (muscle mass) losses experienced by most dieters, this makes *keeping* weight off a *near-impossibility.*

- In many instances, after each diet, *more weight is regained than was lost dieting.* This is again caused by the metabolic reduction that occurs with dieting, which also results in fatigue, confusion, intolerance to cold temperatures, sleep disturbances, depression, and a host of other ailments. And of course, the primary problem with dieting is that the weight usually does not stay off.

  This is not "your fault". It's the whole concept of dieting that is at fault.

- Dieting even increases the activity of certain enzyme systems in the body that work to *increase the rate of fat storage.* Your body, in effect, becomes a "fat storing machine", zealously guarding its precious fat stores in the face of what it believes is a state of imminent starvation. It doesn't know you're trying to lose weight! Quite literally, **dieting makes you fatter!** Remember that dieting can also make you fatter by decreasing lean body mass (muscles), which further pushes the balance in favor of fat, making it harder to lose weight each time.

- The use of pre-packaged, highly processed, dehydrated, unnatural, unhealthful, nutritionally empty, and environmentally polluting "meals" or "meal substitutes" can lead to more than just a failure to keep lost weight off. The risk of serious gallbladder, kidney, gastrointestinal, heart, metabolic and other diseases is believed to be significantly elevated in people undergoing rapid calorie-restriction-generated weight loss programs, *especially* those using "meal substitutes" or "meal replacements". Dieting can kill you!

- Today's commercial weight loss programs take full advantage of these well-known, scientifically proven facts. They continue to market their prepackaged, nutritionally empty foods, or worse — "meal-replacements" and so-called "diet shakes" and "diet bars" that are supposed to substitute for one, two, and sometimes all three daily meals. They know that most of their customers today will probably be customers again tomorrow because most will gain all their weight back (and then some). They *depend* on this, as part of their plan. All such products and all such companies should be shunned.

If you are overweight, and/or tired all the time, if you are in pain, sick too often, or otherwise unhealthy — *something* needs to change. It cannot be a thoughtless, quick fix. It must be a *permanent, healthful* solution. In other words, BioSlim.

BOTTOM LINE: *Forget dieting,* as most of us have come to know it. Never "go on a diet" again.

TWELVE

THE BIOSLIM FOOD PLAN
Eat All the Real, <u>Good</u> Food You Want
ᘂᘀ

With the BioSlim program, *you* will choose foods to include in your permanent, lifetime Food Plan. Studies have shown that when people choose their own foods, as opposed to trying to follow a predetermined program, they are more likely to *like it,* and more likely to *stick to it.*

Two concepts here are central to the BioSlim philosophy:

1) *Individual choice is vital.* Using the BioSlim guidelines, <u>you</u> choose what you're going to eat. We will not give you a menu plan you must follow for a week, a month, or even one day. What would be the point? How long are you likely to follow our menu plan? In order to make this a permanent solution, you must make permanent changes. Obviously. So *you* decide how you're going to eat. But in designing your personal Food Plan, do follow the principles we will outline in the following pages regarding which foods to choose.

2) *It is important that you like what you're doing.* If you don't, if you're unhappy, you won't be able to keep it up. You'll end up struggling, and will probably "give it up" many times along the way. The BioSlim program strives to help you find a food plan that is at once healthful, weight regulating, and *satisfying.* Sure, there will be some foods you will have to give up. Do it gladly, knowing that each and every one of them is not only fattening, but *destructive to your health* and would shorten your life if you kept eating it. No food is "off

the list" if it is healthful. The only ones proscribed are the ones that carry a double jeopardy: <u>they increase your body fat and worsen your health</u>. This should make it much easier to stick to the right stuff.

Later in this chapter we will review specific foods you may include in your food plan and the ones you should avoid. But now, let's review the central principles you should use in choosing foods to include in your new, permanent Food Plan, and in determining how you eat them. With these principles and criteria in mind, you can judge any food, anytime, anywhere, and decide whether it is or is not a fitting candidate.

REMEMBER: Think of food as *important.* It is. What you eat directly affects your health and how long you're going to live. With this in mind, approach every food decision as something to think carefully about. Once you make your decision, you won't have to make it again. Soon, you'll have identified the foods you want to include and exclude, and from that point on you will never have to think much about how you eat.

This is the goal: to stop the unhappiness and deprivation, and to make this process you are in *enjoyable* and fun.

ESSENTIAL PRINCIPLES OF THE BIOSLIM FOOD PLAN:

1) AVOID ADDED FATS AND OILS

The primary BioSlim Food Plan principle

This is the most important rule to remember, and it cannot be overemphasized. The words *"added fats and oils"* have a very specific and special meaning here, namely: **those unnatural fats and oils that *humans* manufacture, process, and add to the food you eat.** There are no such things as *pure* or *added* fats and oils in nature. They just don't exist! NATURE makes corn and peanuts... HUMANS make corn and peanut oils, margarine and deep-fried food. NATURE creates soybeans... HUMANS manufacture soy oil and mayonnaise. It is extremely important to avoid

ALL these added fats and oils, not just because they'll make you fat but also because they'll make you **sick**.

Added fats and oils have been clearly linked to such serious problems as breast and colon cancers, heart disease, and other illnesses. These are some of today's most deadly diseases. You really should think of the appearance issue, then, as not the most important reason to avoid added fats and oils. The most important reasons have to do with your health, and *how long you're going to live!* And yes, of course, these manufactured additions to your food will certainly also make you fat.

SO REMEMBER, **NO ADDED FATS AND OILS!** That includes margarine, mayonnaise, butter, oily salad dressings, chips of all kinds (unless they're baked), fried foods, french fries, cream cheese, ice cream, lard, and others. And if you don't like salads without dressing—try lemon juice and seasoning salt. It's delicious! Or... try any of the *oil-free* salad dressings now widely available, and especially, any of the extraordinarily delicious, healthful salad dressing recipes in the *BioSlim CookBook,* the companion to this book.

Note that of all the added fats and oils, products like margarine, mayonnaise and all likewise *hydrogenated* or *heated* fats and oils are the worst of the bunch. They are high in *trans* fats, substances that form when fat or oil is heated or heavily processed, which are directly implicated in the etiology and exacerbation of cardiovascular disease and cancer. Avoid these "foods" at all costs.

2) TRY TO EAT REAL, RECOGNIZABLE FOOD
The Ultimate Criterion

This second general criterion for judging food is similar to the first, but broader. Basically, it is: "Look at what you're about to eat, and consider whether you *recognize* what it is". You can tell what a vegetable, a fruit, or even a piece of meat is, and you know where it came from. But if food comes in a box, a can, or a package—beware. **READ LABELS!** The fact that you do not recognize something you're about to eat is like a warning sign telling you to **READ THE LABEL,** and to be on the lookout for possibly harmful ingredients.

In particular, besides avoiding all added fats and oils, you should try mightily to avoid refined sugar. It's in a lot of foods, mostly of the junk variety. If you see it on a label, you'd do well to skip that product.

In general, imagine yourself away from civilization, in a completely natural setting: Foods that you would find in that setting are generally OK. Otherwise—if it comes in a can or box, or is a powder or a "shake"—be careful. And if you cannot understand the label, be extra careful.

The BEST possible foods to eat are green vegetables: eat all you want of them (within reason, of course).

There are, in fact, several vegetables that actually use up more energy getting digested than they bring to your body. The digestion of any food requires an expenditure of energy by the body. Once the food is digested, it releases its own stored energy in the form of calories, which are then either used ("burned") or stored, mostly as fat. Sometimes, the number of calories in a food is lower than the number of calories it takes to digest it. The act of eating, for example, celery or cucumber, can be a weight losing proposition all by itself—without exercise or anything! Now isn't that interesting...?

Vegetables whose digestion can use more calories than they contain include:

ALFALFA SPROUTS	CUCUMBER
BEET GREENS	EGGPLANT – *(a close call)*
BROCCOLI – *(a close call)*	ENDIVE
CABBAGE	GARLIC
CAULIFLOWER – *(close call)*	LETTUCE
CELERY	MUSHROOMS
CHARD, SWISS	PEPPERS – *(a close call)*
CHIVES	RADISHES

SEAWEEDS – *(all kinds)*
SPINACH
TOMATO – *(a close call)*

TURNIP GREENS
WATER CHESTNUTS
WATERCRESS

3) EAT IN CORRECT BALANCE

Matching carbohydrates to proteins; fats per Principle #1

Optimally, you should eat, by weight or equivalent volumes, approximately as much high-protein food as you do high-carbohydrate food.

Protein is defined in the *Nutrition: The Key to Health* chapter below. It is found in high percentages in lean meat, poultry, eggs (esp. egg whites!), low-fat fish, soy products, spirulina, low fat dairy products, etc. Your best bet is to find nearly-*pure* protein foods to supplement your other food. Then, in any given meal, if you feel you have not eaten sufficient protein for the carbohydrates you've had, simply eat one of these nearly-pure protein foods to make up the difference. Examples include:

- Fat-free deli slices: available in your local supermarket, the best of these are made from chicken or turkey. They are virtually pure protein.
- Egg white: pure protein. Prepare as hard-boiled, or as omelets (yolks removed).
- Fat-free or low-fat **soy** deli slices, hot dogs, sausage, etc.: available in health stores and some supermarket. These are your best choices, because not only are they almost pure protein, they also have *fiber* in them! Unlike all animal products, these soy-based foods do have the fiber your digestive system needs to operate smoothly. And they are delicious too! Excellent choices, all around.

So... a quick meal could comprise: fat-free deli slices (regular or soy), as many as you like, plus asparagus (canned or fresh) and other vegetables.... and off you go. Quick, nutritious, easy.

Carbohydrates are also defined in the *Nutrition: The Key to Health* chapter below. The highest levels of carbohydrates, and the worst offenders when it comes to balancing your foods, are foods made from flour. Any grain is high in carbohydrates. Flour products are particularly concentrated. This includes breads, pasta, cakes, pancakes, etc.

Sugar is also a carbohydrate. Anything sweet is likely to be carbohydrate-rich (unless made with sugar substitutes, of course). Sugar of any kind should be avoided, though fructose (fruit sugar) is absorbed much slower than sucrose (table sugar), and is therefore a better choice (lower insulin response, less likely to convert to fat).

Other examples of foods to avoid because they are too concentrated in carbohydrates include: potato, corn, banana, carrot and fruit juices (which should always be diluted at least in half with water).

Regarding **fats**, the third constituent of food: do not worry about it. All you need remember is to avoid added fats. That's it. Don't count fat grams, don't worry over what percentage of your calories are coming from fat—do nothing but *avoid all added fats*. That, Principle #1 of BioSlim, is the key to handling the fats in your diet.

Balancing your food intake correctly, as described here, will aid your body in achieving the metabolic balance it needs to normalize itself. Most Americans eat way too many carbohydrates, and are therefore susceptible to the problems of chronically high insulin levels, obesity, and all the other problems that come with an unhealthy system. **Balance** is the key.

If in doubt, err on the side of more proteins. Excess carbohydrates will wreck your success. Excess protein will do little harm, and may even help a bit.

Note: If the carbohydrate food you are eating is "puffed" in any way—as are most breakfast cereals, cake and even bread—volume judgments must be tempered by some estimate of actual weight.

Note: As mentioned previously, if your blood tests show a high level of *serum triglycerides*, it may well be a sign that you are intolerant to carbohydrates, and that you MUST cut back as much as possible on sugars, all grain products, and the other high-carb items described above, if you are to succeed in losing weight and normalizing your system.

4) EAT SMALLER MEALS MORE FREQUENTLY; MEAL TIMING

Lighter, more frequent eating instead of 1 or 2 large meals a day

Many people eat just one significant meal a day, usually dinner. This is not at all a good idea. It means that you are going hungry during most of the day, and that you will digest poorly, eat too much, probably sleep badly and... gain weight faster. Studies have showed that eating a given amount of food *distributed* through the day will result in less weight gain than eating the same amount all in one meal. This may have to do with the blood sugar, and hence insulin, roller coaster your body is on when you eat your whole day's food in one meal. It is not healthful, and it is likely to lead to obesity.

Timing of meals: Try to eat some food every 5 hours or so. *Distribute* your daily food intake over several meals, with most of it at breakfast and lunch. One study showed that when two comparable groups of people eat the same number of calories but on different schedules, the group that eats one large meal per day gains weight and feels worse, while the group that spreads its calories throughout the day feels better and gains no weight.

Other studies indicate that when food is eaten late in the day, weight is gained as compared to no weight gain when the *same food* is eaten earlier in the day. Therefore:

LARGEST MEAL: Lunch

SMALLEST MEAL: Dinner

MODERATE OR LARGER MEAL: Breakfast

This is the optimal way to arrange your days. The typical large dinner with which most people are familiar is problematic because (a) the natural daily rhythms of the body are such that evening is when it is preparing for rest, not a large meal; and (b) food eaten late in the day will more likely be converted into body fat which, once stored, comes off much slower, and with much greater difficulty than it came on. Eat light dinners—salad, perhaps a soup and a small side dish. Not much more.

The absolute *worst* time to eat is at or near bedtime. Those late-night snacks are a terrible idea because the food eaten within two or three hours of sleep will almost *certainly* be converted to body fat.

For **breakfast,** follow your body's signals. Optimally, you should eat a solid breakfast, high in protein (like spirulina!). But if you're not very hungry in the morning, it's OK to eat lighter. However, you should always eat *some* breakfast! It sets the tone for your whole day. (See *Spirulina For Breakfast?* below.)

Lunch is the perfect time to eat your largest meal of the day, if you have one. There's plenty of time left to burn it off, and the satiety will probably last well into dinner time, thereby helping to keep dinners small.

ABOUT THE *SUPER BIOSLIM* PLAN

This is a new addition to BioSlim. It includes a more intensive Food Plan, and is designed for use by those individuals who do not readily find success under the standard BioSlim program. Super BioSlim is not designed to be adopted permanently. It is, rather, a limited-term way to "get the ball rolling" in terms of weight loss and overall results. Once success is achieved using Super BioSlim, a return to some form of the standard BioSlim program is highly recommended. Some individuals eventually settle on a *combination* of the two plans that they believe they can maintain permanently—which is perfectly OK. The key word is: *permanent.*

Super BioSlim can be used to achieve very rapid weight loss by anyone, without even trying the standard BioSlim plan. It is recognized that some people will do this. If you are one of them, remember that Super BioSlim is not meant as a permanent solution to weight control. Consider it a "quick fix". A *permanent* program must still be adopted if you are to avoid the infamous "yo-yo" phenomenon. That permanent program can be the regular BioSlim plan, or some combination with Super BioSlim.

Super BioSlim is described in detail in the *Appendix*.

FOOD RATING GUIDE

Now we will review specific foods. They are categorized for you here, but please take the opportunity to apply the BioSlim Principles just described to each of these foods, so that you may see how and why the process works.

Wherever possible, foods are listed by category. Since *you* will be choosing foods to include in your new Food Plan, this is done to make your choices wider and easier; any food that logically belongs in the same category as those listed here may be treated in the same manner. The listings, then, are here merely as examples, rather than as foods you *must* eat.

Note that the grading system is flexible. Not every food in the "may eat at will" section should really be eaten at will: the point is that these foods are considered both healthful and weight-control-friendly, and may be consumed in a *reasonable* manner without thought of control. The "2-3 times per week" foods are also in a flexible category, in that the frequency of ingestion may be adjusted to individual needs and lifestyles: you could eat these foods more or less frequently, within reason, as you will decide.

The key issues remain those embodied in the Principles of the BioSlim Food Plan described above. The rest should be made to fit your particular needs *by you*—not by us with some arbitrary "diet" that we lay out for you (so that you can abandon it one day!) Let us avoid that at all costs.

Do it the way *you* like it, using the following lists and categories as guidelines.

NOTE: "Cheating" (or "indulging") is discussed at the end of this chapter.

Food Rating Guide

THE RIGHT STUFF - I
FOODS THAT MAY BE CONSUMED AT WILL, WITHIN REASON

- **Vegetables** – especially the **green** ones, which are the best. Seaweeds are particularly excellent choices. Be aware that it is possible to transform any vegetable dish from very healthful to very *un*healthful by throwing in added fats or oils, like butter, margarine, or oil itself.

    NOTE: See the information above under *Eat in Correct Balance* regarding potatoes, corn, carrots. These foods are quite high in carbohydrates and need to be balanced as above.

- **Fat-free or low-fat meat, poultry and deli slices** – those packaged fat-free chicken or turkey slices in the deli section are the best choices here. These are virtually pure protein, and may be used at will to balance out carbohydrate (flour products, sugar, etc.) intake.

- **Fat-free or low-fat soy products** – such as: deli slices, hot dogs, sausage rolls, hamburger blend, etc. These are soy products made to taste just like the real thing. Why bother? Because these products are far more healthful than their animal-based counterparts. They contain *fiber*, which no animal product does. And they are plant-based, and hence have none of the accumulated toxins, antibiotics and hormones animal products (meat) can have. All in all, these are your best choices for solid high-protein sources.

- **Eggs and especially egg whites** – egg whites are pure protein, and may be eaten at will. Use them to balance any excess carbohydrate intake. May be prepared in any manner, such as hard-boiling, frying or poaching (boiling is best).

    Eggs have historically been much maligned because of the issue of cholesterol (see the *Cholesterol* section of the *Medical Considerations* chapter above). In fact, studies where people have eaten up to 18 eggs per week indicate that eggs do *not* cause cholesterol to rise. The whole idea that eating eggs will cause blood cholesterol levels to rise because there is a significant amount of cholesterol in them is simplistic and false. In fact, eating eggs can even help levels *drop*, depending on the rest of the diet. Eating cholesterol has never been shown to cause cholesterol levels to rise, since most of the body's cholesterol is made internally, mostly in the liver. The primary factors controlling cholesterol levels are heredity and overall nutritional and physical well-being (again, see the *Medical Considerations* chapter above).

Eggs contain the most perfect protein available in food. They are also loaded with vitamins, minerals, lecithin, etc., with a moderate amount of fat. They contain no fiber, however, like all animal products.

Eggs may be eaten up to approximately 6-8 per week, though more may be eaten if you determine that you can tolerate them.

Note: Do not ruin eggs by frying them in oil, or by melting cheese on or in them.

As above, egg *whites* may be eaten at will, in virtually any amounts. The whites contain pure protein, with no fat and no carbohydrates.

- **Beans and peas** (in moderation) – includes soybeans, kidney beans, lima beans, green peas, etc. These are terrific sources of protein (especially soybeans), fiber, and other nutrients.

- **Soups** – this is not really a category on its own, but is mentioned because, made properly—with no oil added, and no junk food thrown in—soups can be delicious, filling, *and* healthful all at the same time. See the *BioSlim CookBook* for the best soup recipes in the world (my opinion, of course).

- **Fat-free or low-fat milk, cheese and yogurt** – Fat *free* products are best. Even low-fat milk is a relatively *high* fat food. (Because most of milk is water, the fat in it equals a high percentage of its *dry* weight, even in so-called "low-fat" milk products.)

See *Colitis* under *Medical Considerations* above for more important information on milk products. If you are not one of the *billions* of people on the planet who are sensitive or allergic to milk, then these products are OK.

Note: if you *are* sensitive to milk you should also avoid yogurt, because the substance you may be most sensitive to—the milk protein *casein*—is present in yogurt in the same manner and amount as it is in regular milk. Lactose, the sugar in milk that so many people are intolerant of ("lactose intolerance"), is present in far *lower* quantities in yogurt as opposed to milk due to the lactose-digesting action of the bacteria that ferment milk into yogurt. But remember: lactose intolerance is only one form of milk sensitivity. The other form, typically an *allergy* to milk protein, is not ameliorated by the fermentation process, nor can it be treated with lactase pills.

If you eat yogurt, get the non-fat variety. And get it without sugar and the other junk that is often thrown in "for taste".

Also: Fresh, real yogurt contains beneficial bacteria (*lactobacillus*). Frozen yogurt, on the other hand, does not qualify as true yogurt, as it has no live beneficial bacteria in it. It is often not much more than colored milk and sugar. Avoid it.

- **Lemon juice** – used with vegetable seasoning salt – makes a great, non-fat salad dressing.
- **Apple cider vinegar** – great on salads. Healthful.
- **Water and herbal teas** – the best herbal teas are chamomile and peppermint, and there are many other delicious ones for you to enjoy. (Water is discussed later.)

THE RIGHT STUFF - II
FOODS FOR MODERATE CONSUMPTION (2-3 TIMES/WEEK)

- **Fish and Seafood** – are theoretically quite healthful. They generally contain plenty of high quality protein and moderate amounts of healthful oils. The concern here relates to contamination. It has been determined recently that every fish in every ocean in the world is now contaminated in some way with chemical and/or radioactive pollutants. This astounding, profoundly disturbing fact should lead you to think twice about the fish and seafood you eat. Choose fish from relatively clean areas, far from industrial shores (e.g., Alaskan fish are considered excellent choices). And be sure the fish you do eat is fresh; it is very easy to get spoiled or partially spoiled fish in restaurants and markets.

- **Poultry** – white meat, if possible. The dark meat has a significantly higher fat content (fatty tissue is where most environmental toxins, antibiotics and hormones are found). The fat in chicken is of the saturated variety, and less healthful than that found in fish. Remove skins before eating. Like all animal products, try to keep this down to twice or thrice weekly.

- **Lean meat** – occasional consumption (if _lean_) is OK. Not recommended, though, for reasons related to health. See below.

- **Tofu** and related foods – Tofu is a soybean derivative, aka "soy cheese". It is quite healthful, though low in fiber and *not* low in (natural) fat. Occasional use is no problem. Note that tofu is basically tasteless; it typically acquires the flavor of any food with which it is prepared.

- **Wheat-based breads** –the most common bread ingredient. Wheat is a highly concentrated carbohydrate source, and should be eaten in moderation and always balanced with protein. It is also a very common allergen (allergy-causing substance). And unfortunately, most breads made with wheat are made with processed white flour. Even so-called "wheat bread" is usually white flour with a little coloring or bran thrown in. When you do eat wheat-based bread, eat only those whose label reads *100% whole wheat*. If possible, try to alternate with breads made of other grains, such as true whole rye, rice, millet, corn, and others. These alternative breads are generally available in specialty shops or health stores.

Best advice: Get your carbohydrates from vegetables, some fruit, and whatever flour is used in cooking your food. It is a waste of carbohydrate "space" to eat bread very often.

- **Occasional other (*whole*) grains** – in approximately descending order of healthfulness, examples are: millet, quinoa, buckwheat, brown rice, amaranth, corn, whole wheat. "Whole" is the key here. Most grains, especially wheat, are highly processed by the time you get them in the store. White flour, or the deceptively named "wheat flour", is ground wheat from which virtually all the essential nutrition and fiber are removed. "Enriched" flour is the same, except that a small handful of vitamins are thrown in to keep it legal. White rice is similarly processed and nutritionally defective. *Whole* grains, by contrast, are for the most part in their natural state. If you are going to eat grains, stick to the *whole* ones.

    NOTE: Grains are very high-carbohydrate foods and should be eaten in moderation. Best advice: don't waste your carbohydrate "space" on too many grains.

- **Occasional fruit** – enjoy seasonal fruit from time to time. Fruits are loaded with nutrients and fiber; they have a *cleansing* effect on the body. However, they tend to be sweet: high in sugar. Balance these sugar carbohydrates as above.

    Fruit *juices* are a whole different matter. They should be held to a minimum. If drunk, they should be *diluted* first with water. The reason for this is that fruit juices contain highly concentrated amounts of sugar. Yes, it's more healthful sugar than the white table variety, but it's still sugar, and there's just too much of it all in one place in fruit juices. Note that *juice* does not exist in nature. Nature intended for fruit to be eaten whole. It is safe to assume that the wholesale juicing, pasteurizing and packaging of fruit was not part of the plan. If you love juice and must have it, do dilute it first with water, at least 50:50. It actually tastes *better* this way! Also: drinking plenty of water during the day should reduce your craving for juice. And if you do indulge, try to get juice fresh-squeezed whenever possible. And *then* dilute it.

- **Occasional nuts and seeds** – nuts and seeds contain several healthful constituents, including protein, minerals, vitamins, and healthful, essential oils. Since the oil in nuts and seeds is not "added" by humans, it is technically OK under the BioSlim plan. But watch it—they still *do* contain lots of calories, and should therefore be eaten in strict moderation.

    If you like nut (or seed) butters—peanut butter, almond butter, tahini (sesame seed butter) etc.—here's a trick you can use to significantly lower their fat contents. First, do NOT get the homogenized nut butters typically sold in supermarkets. They often have *oil added to them,* which is incredible and ridiculous considering how much natural oil they already contain. Get only the all-natural nut butters that *separate.* You should be able to see the oil separated from and layered on top of the nut butter. Let the jar stand undisturbed in a cupboard for two to three days, so that the oil separates fully. Then, gently open the jar and *pour off the oil layered on top.* Using a paper towel, wipe off any excess oil lying on top that may not have poured off completely. The butter that remains after pouring should have about 1/2 the oil content it normally has, with no change in flavor. And: practice moderation here!

- **Diluted fruit juices** – See note on *Fruits* above. Instead of fruit juices, try some good herbal teas instead, like peppermint, chamomile or any of the fruity ones. Or try a flavored, unsweetened mineral water; it contains no sugar—just calorie-free flavor extract—and is very refreshing.

FOODS TO AVOID
IN APPROXIMATE DESCENDING ORDER OF NEED TO AVOID

- **MOST IMPORTANT! AVOID ALL FATS and OILS that are ADDED to food.** EXAMPLES: margarine, butter, oil, oily salad dressings, mayonnaise, fried foods, lard, cream cheese, cheeses, etc. These so-called "foods" will both ruin your figure and shorten your life. Pretend they don't exist.

- **ICE CREAM** – *extremely* bad idea. Ice cream is basically fat, refined sugar, flavoring (usually artificial), assorted texturizing chemicals (including one commonly used in auto *antifreeze*) and preservatives. Not exactly a health-building food. Ice cream is one of the worst foods you can eat.

- **ALL CHIPS** – e.g., *potato chips, corn chips,* etc. These are nothing more than carriers of heated oil. Zero nutrition, maximum harm. And to top it off, they are very high in concentrated carbohydrates too. Avoid!

- **REFINED (WHITE) SUGAR** – has been linked to many diseases and disorders—everything from dental decay to heart disease. It comes in many forms and with many names, including: sugar, cane sugar, corn syrup, sucrose, dextrose, maltose, saccharose, invert sugar, etc. Avoid 'em all.

- **CANDIES AND COOKIES** – most are not a good idea, though some, made with natural cane extract, honey, and whole grain flour, are OK for *occasional* indulgence.

- **REFINED (WHITE) FLOUR** – is very common and hard to avoid. Most people eat some of this every day of their lives. The problem: it is nutritionally empty due to the processing applied to it, and extremely high in concentrated carbohydrates. White flour is also devoid of fiber, a true travesty of what nature intended. It is likely to both cause weight gain and contribute to disease (like diabetes, heart disease, colon cancer, etc.) Stick to whole wheat and other whole grains.

- **PEANUT BUTTER** – unless prepared as described above under *Nuts and Seeds*. In any event, regardless of method of preparation, strict moderation is advised.

- **ALCOHOL** – some use is OK. If you do indulge, stick to the wines, which can actually be healthful, *in moderation*. Alcohol is a fuel, and will contribute to obesity if ingested in excess — in addition to ruining your liver. (Note: alcohol has been shown to slow fat metabolism. Hence: moderation!)

- **CHOCOLATE** – OK, OK... if you must, once in a while – you can cheat a little... Cocoa powder, without the oils and sugars usually added to chocolate, is the preferred form. Pure cocoa can actually aid weight loss, as it contains certain enzyme-active substances that can help the body burn fat. As is often the case in our society, the problem is not the natural product, but the way it is prepared — with either the bad stuff added to the natural product or the good stuff removed. Read labels carefully to avoid all the junk usually thrown into chocolate products (mostly lots of fat and sugar).

- MOST **CEREALS** – are usually loaded with refined WHITE SUGAR and WHITE FLOUR (see above). These are always very high in concentrated carbohydrates, so be careful here. Also, try eating cereal with vanilla, chocolate, or carob low-fat soy-milk, instead of regular cow's milk.

- Packaged **PUDDINGS** – are mostly chemicals in a box. Read the label carefully. You'll probably want to throw it away.

- **SOFT DRINKS** – are mostly sugar plus artificial colorings and flavorings. Most do not qualify as real food. Recommended alternatives: flavored, calorie-free mineral water, herbal teas, diluted juices (in moderation).

- Assorted **JUNK FOOD** – too numerous to list. This includes everything made of processed, unnatural, unrecognizable products. You know it when you eat it. Right?

- **RED MEAT** – is usually very high in saturated fats. The more tender the meat, the higher the fat content. You cannot always see the fat because it is *marbled* in the meat.

    Meat has zero fiber. It generally comes from animals that are fed special drugs to make them fatter, as well as antibiotics, hormones, and often, pesticide-laden feed. Many of the chemical substances used on animals are present in trace amounts in red meat, usually stored in the fat.

Yes, meat falls within the BioSlim Food Plan because it is a whole, real, recognizable food, and contains no *added* fats. But due to the way meat is produced these days, and due to the fact that it is, nevertheless, high in fat and less than optimally healthful, it is recommended that red meat be either avoided altogether or eaten infrequently. By eating less meat, you'll also be helping the environment, as it takes many times more food and water to produce meat than it does plant-derived food; you'll be saving precious natural resources, and helping to reduce environmental pollution.

SALT

Many people ask this question: how much salt can I eat if I'm trying to lose weight. Answer: as much as you would any other time. It has no effect on your loss of fat. Reducing salt intake *will* however temporarily cause more water to leave your body. You may *think* you're losing fat, when in fact you are losing water—which always comes back. As a result of excess water loss, you could get dehydrated: dizzy when standing, weak, constipated, tired, sickly and having heart palpitations. Your best bet is to not worry about salt unless you have a kidney or high blood pressure problem, or your doctor tells you to cut back.

ABOUT WATER

It is important to maintain adequate water intake at all times. When you're trying to lose weight, it is doubly important. Water can help give you a feeling of fullness and reduce the amount of food you eat. And it is vital for flushing out unwanted toxins and metabolic byproducts.

Note that thirst is often mistaken for hunger! Often, we eat because we feel the need for something in our mouths. Yet it is water we crave, without knowing it.

Many people live their lives, daily, *chronically dehydrated!* Always "dry" internally. The negative effects are many: constipation, dry skin, rashes, aches and pains, arthritis, even cardiovascular problems can ensue. It is *essential* to give your body the water it needs every day to maintain good health!

The correct amount of water to drink per day varies with each individual. Eight cups is a fair average. Juices, coffee, milk — all do not count fully; figure ½ cup for each cup you drink of these beverages (unless they are diluted, of course).

Tap water can be so loaded with chemicals as to be malodorous. Boiling water can get rid of some of the chemicals, such as chlorine, but may actually *increase* the concentration of some pollutants (because the water evaporates away, leaving these pollutants in the now more concentrated solution).

Best advice: drink bottled spring or mineral water or distilled water. Any of these is better than the chemistry lab that comes out of many of our faucets.

COFFEE

The stimulatory effect of caffeine on the body is literally drug-like, since caffeine is a bona fide drug. It can exacerbate headaches and ulcer disease (see *Headaches* and *Ulcers* under *Medical Considerations* above). The other side of this coin is that coffee can help with weight loss, in that it is a mild stimulant and may help with fat burn-off. The best advice about coffee is: don't rely on it. Moderate use is not usually a problem, but if you're hooked on 5–6 cups a day, you would do well to reduce your dependency. (You know you're dependent if you get a headache {daily, for up to 5-7 days} when you try to quit.)

FOOD PREPARATION

This subject could fill a book all by itself. And it does: the *BioSlim CookBook*, to which the reader is referred for a wealth of information on foods, their definitions and preparation. You will find it highly entertaining and informative. Every recipe there is gourmet quality, yet approved for healthfulness and weight control—without sacrificing taste in any way. Have fun with it!

SPIRULINA FOR BREAKFAST?

Some individuals who are not "morning people" choose to eat only a *power food* in the morning—a "shake", if you will. BioSlim does not recommend the use of any commercially processed powdered foods or shakes. There is, however, one "power food" that we recommend enthusiastically: *Spirulina,* which is not processed at all, but is, rather, a microscopic plant (actually a *blue-green algae*) that comes as a dry powder or in tablets or capsules.

Spirulina is uniquely high in digestible protein (it is about 70% protein—higher that meat!), beta carotene (vitamin A precursor), iron (rare for a plant product), and vitamin B12 (virtually unheard of in a plant product). It is the perfect power food, as it is all-natural, coming to us pretty much as it grows in nature (except that it is dried, of course). Note that *chlorella,* another more expensive blue-green algae, is also excellent.

Spirulina has only one thing wrong with it: most people think it tastes *awful*. The best way to prepare it is to add the powder to a running blender which has in it diluted fruit or vegetable juice in sufficient quantity to create a drinkable liquid blend *and* kill that wonderful spirulina flavor. (OK, I admit: I hate the flavor. But I still drink it down most every morning!)

Tablets and capsules are fine, but they are less digestible, and it is unlikely that you could take enough of them to matter. You would have to take approximately 40 pills to equal two tablespoons of powdered spirulina, about 60 to equal three. Clearly, this is simply not feasible for most people.

If you decide to use spirulina (or chlorella), start with just ½ teaspoon in the blender and work your way up to 2–3 tablespoons over a period of 10–14 days. This will help you avoid any digestive difficulties that sometimes come with the introduction of such a completely new, powerful food.

From personal experience, I can assure you, spirulina is a great way—the best way—to start your day. You'll have lots of energy, your appetite will be gone, and you'll feel great that day. Try it for breakfast!

WHEN TO EAT; WHEN TO STOP

It is instructive to note how naturally thin people eat. Their way happens to match the way primitive man ate—a good indication that it is how nature intended for us to eat. Naturally thin people:

1) Eat only when they are hungry; and

2) Stop eating when they are no longer hungry.

Though this may seem simple and obvious at first glance, it is, in fact, the hardest thing for most people to do in the area of food.

Most of us have been conditioned to eat when it's time to eat: lunch time, dinner time, breakfast. But it is far more natural to *eat when you're hungry*. *Truly* hungry, not just craving food. As much as possible, try to follow this simple, albeit difficult ideal of eating.

The second timing principle is even harder. Most of us are taught in childhood to *finish* what's in front of us.

Eat! Children are starving in Somalia/Bosnia/Rwanda wherever...

That may be true, but it is no reason to stuff yourself. Childhood lessons are not always good ones. The most *natural* way to eat is to *stop when you're no longer hungry.* That means you stop even if 95% of the food is still left on your plate or if only 5% is left. It doesn't matter. The amount of food on the plate is of no importance; it is completely arbitrary and irrelevant to your body's needs. What *is* important is only how you feel. If you're satisfied, if the hunger is gone, *stop*.

If you can master these concepts, you will to a large extent master your nutritional and weight conditions forever. The concepts are simple; we need to act on them.

RESTAURANT EATING

This is a particularly troublesome area. Restaurants, for some unknown reason, love oil. From your local hamburger joint to Chinese food, from Italian to Greek to Indian, and virtually any other restaurant type, they practically *smother* their food with oil and/or cheese. Even simple salads are drowned in truly *ridiculous* amounts of oil. This abuse of oil is the single biggest problem when it comes to eating in restaurants.

But there's more.

Cleanliness is often sub-par. One word of advice: if you're going to be frequenting a restaurant regularly, ask to take a look at the kitchen. Judge for yourself.

Food freshness is another area of concern. Fish, poultry and meat (in descending order) are most likely to be problematic. Be careful. Ask lots of questions, particularly about freshness and oil content. If there is any reason to believe your food is either not fresh or too oily, order something else, or simply leave.

When ordering in a restaurant follow these simple rules:
- Always ask how much oil is in the food you wish to order.
- Insist that the dish(es) you want be made with *no* oil, or at worst, a very small amount.
- Refuse any offer of sprinkled cheese to go over your food.
- Order salads with vinegar dressing only, or lemon wedges that you can squeeze onto the salad. If you must order dressing from the house, get one that *separates,* like vinaigrette, so that you can pour off the oil that floats on top, using only the tasty part below. Best of all: use vinegar plus some salt, or bring your own, healthful salad dressing.
- **Never order anything that is deep fried!** Remember to ask about this, because there are many more foods that are deep fried than is obvious from most menus. For example, Italian restaurants often deep fry their "eggplant parmigiana". You must *ask,* and avoid all foods that are so prepared.
- Avoid creamy foods. Many dishes that are normally prepared with cream are just as tasty without it. Ask the kitchen to prepare it the way you want it.
- Order a salad first, the larger the better, and ask that it be brought out immediately. Avoid the oily/cream dressings, and eat the salad as soon as it comes out. This will help

"take the edge off" your hunger, help you resist the temptation to eat those unhealthful white flour rolls and butter, and get you started in the right direction.
- Try to resist the temptation to order dessert. If you must do so, get one that is as close to "real recognizable food" as you can get. A cup of fruit, or a fruit tart may do (the tart is *not* OK, just a lesser of many evils). In any event, avoid the creamy cakes and pies. Consider them dangerous but tasty poisons to your system.
- In general, do not be afraid to ask for what you want. If they say "no", say "good-bye". There are plenty of restaurants that will be only too happy to accommodate you, so don't put up with anything less than what you know is right for your body.

CHEATING ("INDULGING")

OK, we all know you're going to cheat. Let's get that said and understood. Nobody's perfect. That's why we use that well-worn euphemism, "indulging". The secret of success is: (a) don't do it very often, and (b) when you do cheat, do it in ways that are not so bad for you; i.e., *minimize the damage.*

There is no quota for cheating in the BioSlim program. We urge you to strive for perfection. If you find yourself succumbing once in a while, *consider it cheating,* not your "quota of bad stuff for the week". You should always strive to reject your old, bad ways—to renew your dedication to yourself and to the new body and health you are determined to achieve. Your goal should be to get to the point where cheating is anathema to you, because it means you'll feel physically poor for a while, and because it means you have abused your body.

Now, if you're absolutely determined to do a little cheating, go ahead and do it with something that won't set you back too much. Like some red meat, or thin-crust pizza, or even, occasionally some chips, candy, pie or cookies. Review the order of the *Foods to Avoid* list earlier in this chapter. Do *not* cheat with the first few items in the list. Promise yourself that much.

Remember to balance excess carbohydrates with protein. And don't eat *all* of whatever you're cheating with. Leave some to throw out. That way, you'll get in the habit; someday, you may find yourself throwing it out *before you eat it!*

Note that if you do enough "cheating", you *can* ruin the effect of the BioSlim program. Keep it to a minimum. Don't do it at all if you can help it. If you find you cannot control your impulses to cheat, do the following:

- Read the *Mastering Motivation* chapter later in this book.

- Try reading the *Secret Power Inside You* chapter.

- Read the earlier chapters of this book. Remind yourself of how damaging to your health your actions can be. If you cannot find the motivation to do what has to be done to get thinner, find it instead in the fact that you want to be *healthier*—in the knowledge that eating those foods can damage your body and life in many ways, including causing its premature end. You don't want to wait until it's too late, right?

- Read the *Cravings* chapter below for tips on preventing and controlling those "uncontrollable" urges, including writing down everything you decide to eat *before you eat it*. This alone will often give you time to focus, to realize what you are doing—and change your mind.

- If all else fails, consider hypnotherapy. It's inexpensive and, in qualified hands, highly effective.

THIRTEEN

NUTRITION: THE KEY TO HEALTH
ଓ୫୦

In this chapter, we will first review the general principles of digestion, metabolism and nutrition. We will specifically define the nutritional words: *protein, carbohydrate, fat, vitamin, mineral,* and others. The chapter immediately following will then delve into the use of the BioSlim Formulas: *Vita/Min Plus* and *SlimTone Formula*.

NUTRITION

The term "nutrition" is defined as the relationship of ingested food substances to human health. Nutritional *deficiencies* occur when one or more of the *essential nutrients* are not supplied to the body in adequate amounts. The essential nutrients are: proteins, carbohydrates, fat, water, vitamins and minerals. Each of these is, as the name implies, *essential* to life. The human body can live for extended periods of time with insufficient intake of any of these nutrients except water (without which death may occur in a matter of days). However, though the body may live, it does not necessarily live well. A deficiency of any essential nutrient causes ill health and any number of abnormal symptoms.

To achieve good health, *all* the essential nutrients must be supplied to the body in correct amounts. Their supply does not need to be perfectly accurate, since the body takes what it requires from the nutrients made available to it. In most instances, then, it is OK to supply the body with amounts of vitamins and mineral beyond its true needs, as the body will only use what it needs. This is largely true regarding water as well.

But it is *not* so true of the three major soft-tissue building blocks of the body: the proteins, carbohydrates and fats. These three nutrients all contain *calories,* and function as both building blocks for body tissue, blood, and hormones, and as sources of energy. For the purpose of body repair and maintenance, the human body will use only what it needs of ingested proteins, carbohydrates and fats. The rest is converted to stored energy for future use, and energy is stored in the body mostly in the form of FAT. (There is a minor energy storage in the form of *glycogen,* a substance found in muscle and liver which is used when the body needs energy very rapidly. But glycogen represents just a tiny fraction of the energy stored in the body. The overwhelming majority of it is in the form of body fat.)

This is why overeating causes obesity. And why it is important to feed and treat your body well. In a very real sense, *you are what you eat.* Your body does not function in a vacuum. It needs constant attention and proper feeding if it is to live healthfully and long.

Most diseases can either be completely avoided or made far less damaging with proper nutrition and body care. This includes today's most devastating diseases, such as heart disease, cancer, diabetes, and many others. This is why this book focuses not only on weight control, but on building good health. The two subjects are completely and irrevocably linked, as they both revolve around—and in fact define—the subject of nutrition.

DIGESTION

"Digestion" and "absorption" are the processes by which the body breaks food down into its usable elements, then proceeds to absorb it into the bloodstream.

Digestion begins in the mouth through chewing and the presence of mouth *enzymes.* Enzymes are chemicals that facilitate the breakdown of food and many other chemical reactions in the body. Digestive enzymes are produced in the human body in the salivary glands of the mouth, and in the stomach, the small intestines and the pancreas.

After the mouth, digestion continues in the stomach and the intestines. See figure below for the anatomical details.

Abdominal Digestive Organs

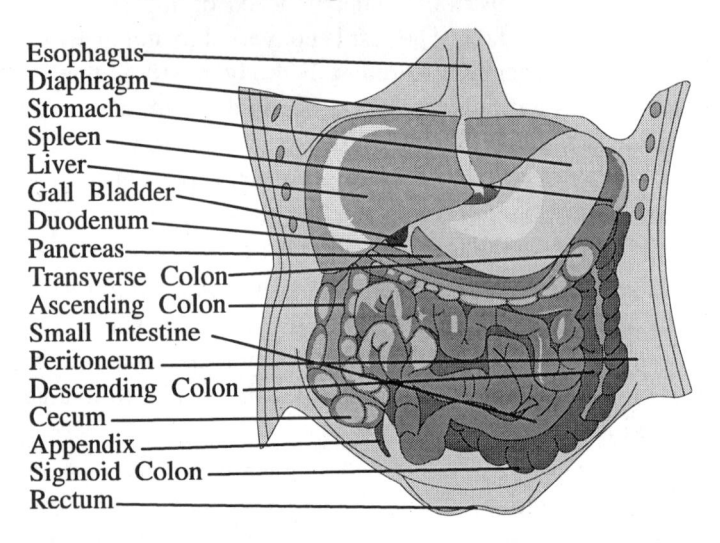

- Esophagus
- Diaphragm
- Stomach
- Spleen
- Liver
- Gall Bladder
- Duodenum
- Pancreas
- Transverse Colon
- Ascending Colon
- Small Intestine
- Peritoneum
- Descending Colon
- Cecum
- Appendix
- Sigmoid Colon
- Rectum

Absorption, the process by which broken-down food is carried into the bloodstream, occurs mostly in the small intestines. The absorbed products—the proteins, carbohydrates, fats, vitamins, minerals, and other substances—are utilized by the body for repair, energy, and for its various nutritional needs.

METABOLISM

Metabolism is defined as the complex of physical and chemical processes involved in the maintenance of life. It comprises the totality of the body's functions. As used in the context of energy usage by the body, the term *metabolic rate* is intended to mean the speed at which the body uses energy—in a sense, how fast the body's "engine" is running.

There are many complex factors affecting metabolic rate—from hormones such as those produced by the thyroid gland, to the body's nutritional status, to what you had for breakfast today and your level of activity (or *in*activity).

Metabolic rate decreases with advancing age.

It is increased during exercise and can be *permanently* increased through a program of regular activity.

Metabolic rate is directly controlled by the thyroid gland, which is why it must be functioning properly for any program of health and body improvement to work. (See *Thyroid gland disease* in the *Medical Considerations* chapter above, and *The Thyroid: Nothing Works If It Does Not* in the *Women: Special Facts and Considerations* chapter below.)

In general, the ingestion of large amounts of fat *reduces* metabolic rate as compared to a similar ingestion of protein or carbohydrates.

Many nutritional factors affect the body's metabolic rate. This is the underlying reason behind the BioSlim Formulas: to provide the body with everything it requires to *normalize* and *optimize* its metabolism.

FOOD COMPONENTS:
WHERE DO CALORIES COME FROM?

There are four basic components of food: protein, carbohydrate, fat, and water. Except, of course, for water, each of these contains stored energy which we call *calories*.

> *NOTE: A calorie is simply a measure of heat energy, defined specifically as the amount of heat needed to raise the temperature of one gram of water 1 degree Celsius, from 14.5°C to 15.5°C. Each pound of body fat represents about 4000 calories, meaning that if a pound of body fat were to be burned as fuel, it would supply enough*

> energy to raise the temperature of 4000 grams (approximately 143 ounces) of water from 14.5°C to 15.5°C.

The chemicals used in processing and packaging food are not counted as they have no nutritive function.

Each of the three non-water, calorie-containing components of food—protein, carbohydrate and fat—has a specific role to play in the health and maintenance of the human body.

Protein

Protein is a very important building block of the body. It is present everywhere in the body, especially muscle tissue, and is vital to the function of every cell. Enzymes and many of the important chemicals found in blood, for example, are formed from certain types of proteins. It is the body's basic building block.

Protein must be eaten for the human body to survive. It is found in high concentrations in most animal-derived foods (meat, fowl, fish, eggs, milk, etc.), as well as in soybean products, spirulina and other blue-green algae, seeds, legumes, beans, nuts, and some vegetables.

One gram of protein contains about 4 calories of energy.

Each protein in the human body is made of building blocks called *"amino acids"*. There are twenty-two amino acids used by the body, of which eight are considered "essential", meaning they must be obtained from external sources—i.e., food—and cannot be made in the body from other substances. The essential amino acids are: Isoleucine, Leucine, Lysine, Methionine, Phenylalanine, Threonine, Tryptophan, and Valine.

[Some of the amino acids have been used in their individually purified form in the nutritional treatment of certain ailments, such as phenylalanine for fatigue and appetite control, tryptophan for insomnia, PMS, depression, and headaches, and taurine for heart disease and seizures. Recently, the U.S. FDA took tryptophan off the market because one manufacturer appears to have produced a tainted product that caused severe illness in several people. The FDA has not yet re-released tryptophan, despite the fact that this is a completely natural, *essential* amino acid (i.e., if you *didn't* eat it in your food, you would die!), which is unfortunate because it is so effective in the treatment of some quite troublesome, otherwise difficult-to-treat ailments. Tryptophan is itself quite harmless, of course.]

During digestion, protein is broken down into small blocks of amino acids, absorbed into the bloodstream, then used in various combinations by the body. If too much protein is consumed, most of the excess is converted into stored energy as fat.

CARBOHYDRATES

Carbohydrates are "energy" foods. Each cell of the body uses some form of carbohydrate as its basic "fuel".

There are two broad categories of carbohydrates: simple, like sugar, and complex, like starch and/or vegetables. Each gram of carbohydrate carries about 4 calories of energy.

Carbohydrates are not strictly essential to life, though it is impossible to eat real food and not eat carbohydrates. The body can create carbohydrates from other sources (protein and fat) when and if it must.

Simple carbohydrates are a quick source of energy. In fact, the substance most commonly used in the bloodstream as fuel for energy is *glucose,* the simplest of sugars used by the body. *Sucrose,* also known as *saccharose,* or simple white table sugar, is a combination of glucose and *fructose,* another simple sugar found commonly in fruit. Eating sucrose causes a very rapid rise in blood sugar, since the process of breaking sucrose down is rapid, as is its absorption into the bloodstream. Unfortunately, this "sugar rush" is short-lived, as blood sugar levels drop dramatically shortly after an initial "high" is achieved.

White table sugar (sucrose) is quite unhealthful, and should be avoided. Note that pure white sugar does not exist in nature. It is entirely a processed product of human intervention, one that the human body finds very difficult to handle healthfully.

Honey consists of a combination of glucose and fructose known as *invert sugar.* It is *not* the same as sucrose, and contains many nutrients which table sugar (sucrose) lacks. As a sweetener, it is therefore somewhat preferred over white sugar. Both, however, will raise insulin levels and interfere with your protein-carbohydrate balance. They must be watched closely.

Complex carbohydrates are found in highest concentration in grains and the flours made from them, plus in some vegetables, beans, and even to some extent in nuts and seeds. Complex carbohydrates are broken down more slowly in the body as compared to the simpler sugars like sucrose. They provide a more stable, steady source of energy, and for the most part do not cause the same harmful effects of white sugar.

Complex carbohydrates do, however, dramatically alter your balance of proteins to carbohydrates. Bread and other flour products are the single most concentrated form of carbohydrate most people consume, and is largely responsible for the obesity of those who are intolerant to it and all who do not control its intake. Beware of eating too many *concentrated* complex carbohydrates.

Excess carbohydrates are stored mostly as fat in the body. (Some carbs are stored as *glycogen,* a rapidly usable form of stored energy found in muscle and liver tissue.) When fat is broken down for energy, as occurs during weight loss, it is converted first back to sugar for use as fuel by the body.

FATS

Fat is a highly concentrated form of energy storage. Each gram of fat carries 9 calories of energy, more than twice that of protein or carbohydrate. This is one reason why it is so important to avoid added fats in the diet under the BioSlim plan. The fats that are *added* to food generally serve no purpose other than to increase the body's storage of fat, something most of us neither need nor want. Note that the term *oil* simply refers to the liquidity of the fat in question; oil is fat that pours.

Fat is important to the body (see Chapter 2, *Why is There Fat?*). It is present in every single living cell and serves to provide the building blocks for many of the body's hormones.

Certain vitamins are *fat-soluble*, and are carried to and stored in the body by use of fat. And, of course, fat is important structurally to the body: it surrounds and holds in place many vital organs, and insulates the body through its presence under the skin.

Also, certain fat constituents called *Essential Fatty Acids* ("EFAs") are, as their name implies, essential to life much as vitamins are. One of these essential fatty acids, *linoleic acid*, is most important, and cannot be manufactured by the body; it must be ingested in food. GLA (*gamma linolenic acid*, an omega-6 fatty acid) and EPA (*eicosapentaenoic acid*, an omega-3 fatty acid) are the two main types of EFAs. If you are supplementing your diet with these, the correct balance is at least 2-3 parts EPA (or even better, 10 parts or more) to one part GLA.

There are two broad categories of ingested fat, *saturated* and *unsaturated,* terms which have to do with basic chemical structure. Saturated fat molecules have less "holes" or "openings" in their chemical structures with which to interact with other molecules (typically oxygen). They are more stable, and are physically harder (less liquid) at room temperature than their unsaturated counterparts. That's why butter and margarine are solid at room temperature, while corn oil is not. The corn oil is far less *saturated* than the butter and margarine.

Saturated fats have developed an unsavory reputation over the past few decades as the culprits behind heart disease, while unsaturated fats have been championed as possibly helping to *prevent* heart disease. The truth of the matter, though, is that for all the focus on this issue, there has been no appreciable change in the incidence of heart disease attributable to it. Eating unsaturated fats such as corn, sunflower, or peanut oil, *does not reduce the incidence of heart disease!* If anything, it <u>*increases*</u> it, due to increases in *trans* fatty acids (see below, and see *Heart Disease* in the *Medical Considerations* chapter above).

Cholesterol is a fat-related substance that has been much maligned in recent years. In fact, there is no evidence to show that eating cholesterol causes heart disease. <u>None</u>. For most people, the amount of cholesterol in the diet bears no relationship to the level of cholesterol in the blood, no relationship to cardiovascular health, and no relationship whatsoever to longevity. (See above under *Cholesterol level, elevated* in the *Medical Considerations* chapter for more information.)

Importantly, research has shown that eating *heated* fats or oils of any kind is terribly damaging to human health, contributing to the evolution of both cancer and heart disease. This is believed to be due to substances called *trans fatty acids* that are formed when fat (or oil) is heated. Most oil is heated during its production. Also, margarine and all other likewise *hydrogenated* fats and oils contain high levels of these harmful *trans fatty acids*. This is one of the most important reasons that all *added* fats are excluded in the BioSlim System: fats added to food are the ones that are typically processed and/or heated.

The fastest way to get fatter is to eat fat. Research shows that given a fixed number of calories to consume, people who eat most of those calories as fat are much more likely to gain weight, i.e. gain body fat, than are people who eat most of those same number of calories as carbohydrates and protein. In other words, weight maintenance is not merely a matter of calorie intake. The *kinds* of calories you eat is key. The more fat you eat, the higher the probability that you will get fatter.

The best way to know your overall fat intake is to calculate the percentage of your daily caloric intake that is derived from fat. This is done by calculating the total intake of calories from fat for the day (or for a specific food) using the fact that there are 9 calories in each gram of fat, then dividing that *fat-calorie* number by the total calories consumed (per day or per specific food).

> If, for example, you are eating something that has 4 grams of fat and a total calorie count of 80, the percentage of total calories that is derived from fat for that food is:
> - 4 times 9 = 36 => total fat-derived calories
> - 36 divided by 80 = 45% => percentage of total calories derived from fat. This is high.

It is best to keep the *average* daily percentage of calories derived from fat below 20%. Individual foods, though, can vary throughout the day.

Under BioSlim, this calculation is unnecessary. Avoiding all *added* fats is the only key principle you need remember.

VITAMINS

Vitamins are organic substances that are considered essential to human health. They are found only in living things. Most vitamins act in concert with various enzymes in the body to accomplish certain chemical goals; many vitamins act as *coenzymes*. Note that many vitamins also function in the body together with certain essential minerals, addressed below.

Daily human requirements of vitamins vary greatly from individual to individual. The government publishes something it calls the RDA, or Recommended Daily Allowance, for *some* vitamins and minerals. This list is: (a) incomplete, in that it totally ignores several well-known nutrients, and (b) wrong. The amounts listed in the RDA are often extremely, even outrageously, low; they *may* be enough to prevent severe full-blown deficiency illness, but they are often very far from the levels the human body needs to achieve a state of optimal health. Those RDA listings on the backs of bottles, then, are of little value, which is why you see so many large percentage numbers in the "%RDA" column on the labels of high quality vitamin formulas. The bottom line on RDAs: you may ignore them.

Can you get enough vitamins in your diet to achieve good health without supplementation? Well yes, maybe, if you grow your own organic produce, live in a stress-free, pollution-free environment, and always eat correctly. Does that sound like you?

The fact is that it is almost *impossible* for the body to get everything it needs from the typical Western diet. During processing, *most* of the micronutrients present in most foods are destroyed. Survey after survey has shown that most Americans are deficient in several essential vitamins and minerals. The concept that you can "just eat right and get everything you need" is therefore quite wrong, and potentially dangerous.

The following is a list of vitamins, their basic properties, and the amounts required by the body.

Vitamin A

This is a *fat soluble* vitamin important to the maintenance of body tissue, mostly the skin and mucous membranes (the internal lining of the body). It is also important to eyesight and some of the basic functions of the body's cells. Note: Studies have found lower levels of vitamin A in overweight individuals as compared to people with normal weight-to-height ratios.

Vitamin A is found in its complete form only in certain animal tissue, mostly in liver products. However, *carotenes* are substances, found in many vegetables, that are converted into vitamin A by the body. Carrots are famous for being high in *beta carotene*, an antioxidant and the best known form of carotene. Virtually all green and yellow vegetables are rich in carotenes.

Vitamin A is stored in the body, mostly in the liver. Like other fat soluble vitamins, it can accumulate in the body, and can even cause negative reactions (reversible toxicity reactions) if taken in great excess over a prolonged period of time. But the amounts that must be ingested in order to cause actual toxicity reactions are huge, and they typically must be consumed for months at a time. Recorded cases of vitamin A toxicity are rare. Vitamin A deficiency, by contrast, is quite common.

Vitamin A intake should normally be between 5,000 and 10,000 I.U. (I.U.=International Units) per day. To optimize absorbability, it is best taken with food.

Beta carotene may be taken in far larger quantities. The body will use what it needs from of the carotenes consumed (mostly in the form of yellow or green vegetables). (Note: too much carotene can cause {reversible} yellowing of the skin called *carotenemia*.)

The B Vitamins

All the B vitamins are *water soluble,* and are not typically stored in the body to any large extent (vitamin B12 is a major exception). There are many B vitamins, together known as the "B complex". They do not require any fat in the diet for absorption.

The B vitamins are essential to proper metabolism and energy utilization by the body. They are necessary to the body's handling of fats, carbohydrates and proteins, and to the maintenance of most body tissues.

B vitamins are very susceptible to destruction by food processing, which is why so many people in Western society are deficient in one or more of them. Contributing to these deficiencies is overexposure to caffeine, cigarettes, pollution, and stress.

Most B vitamins are found in plant-based food, and in certain meats. The major exception to this is B12, which is rarely found in any food that is not of animal origin; this is why vegetarians may be prone to vitamin B12 deficiencies. Note that *spirulina*, described earlier, is one of the few non-animal products that contains significant amounts of vitamin B12.

Since the B vitamins are water soluble, they can be ingested in quite large quantities without toxicity. However, as always, reason must prevail. Vitamin B6, for example, can cause certain transient neurological problems (tingling, numbness) if taken in very large quantities. High-dose niacin can cause liver damage. Remember, *anything,* even *water,* can be toxic if taken in sufficient quantities. A sensible balance is always the best, safest course.

Listed here are the most important B vitamins, their functions and safe dosages. Actual individual requirements vary greatly.

THE B VITAMINS (with safe daily dosage ranges)

B1 (Thiamine)	20 - 100 mg	Energy production. Digestion. Appetite regulation. Mental function.
B2 (Riboflavin)	20 - 100 mg	Energy production. Digestion. Vision. Tissue maintenance.

B3 (Niacin)	25 - 500 mg	Nervous system function. Tissue maintenance. Hormone production. Digestion.
B5 (Pantothenic Acid)	25 - 500 mg	Adrenal function, stress handling. Cellular and energy metabolism. Hormone production. Protection from toxins.
B6 (Pyridoxine) [*Pyridoxal-5'-phosphate* = very high quality form of B6.]	20 - 150 mg	Food metabolism. Energy production. Immune function. Digestion. Cellular function. Hormonal activity.
B12 (cyanocobalamin)	25 - 1000 mcg	Nervous system function. Red blood cell production. Food metabolism.
Biotin	50 - 400 mcg	Food metabolism. Skin, hair and nail health. Aids in utilization of other vitamins.
Folic Acid	200 - 400 mcg (800 mcg in pregnancy)	Red blood cell formation. Protein metabolism. Mental function. Digestion.

Other substances thought to be in the B vitamin family of nutrients include *choline, inositol* and PABA. Deficiencies of these nutrients are rarer than for those listed in the table above.

Folic acid, vitamin B12, biotin, and vitamin B6 are nutrients often found to be deficient in many diets. *All* these nutrients, however, are important. All must be present in correct amounts, continuously throughout life, in order to achieve and maintain good health. Note: All are in the BioSlim Formulas!

Vitamin C *(Ascorbic Acid)*

The most famous and popular of all vitamins, vitamin C is water soluble, and very important to human health. It is thought that large doses of this vitamin may be helpful in reducing the incidence and severity of such diverse diseases as the common cold, cancer, heart disease, tooth decay, and many, many others.

Vitamin C's most important function in the body is in the formation and healing of body tissues. It is also important to the formation of blood cells, and to the proper function of the immune system. It has also been found to help directly in reducing obesity.

Vitamin C is found in most fresh fruits and vegetables. It is often destroyed in food processing. Pasteurized orange juice, for example, has virtually no vitamin C in it, unless it is added after the fact.

Vitamin C in large quantities is not as well absorbed as are smaller quantities. It is best, therefore, to take vitamin C in several smaller doses during the day, as opposed to a single very large dose.

Vitamin C daily dosages range from as little as 100 or 200 mg all the way to 6,000 mg per day, or more. Anything over 5,000 to 6,000 mg per day is likely to cause diarrhea. 500–600 mg per day is a reasonable maintenance dose, but so is 2,000 to 3,000 per day. Individual need is the best guide. Choose the dose that is most consistent with your good health.

The dose included in the BioSlim Formulas is appropriate for most people; additional vitamin C is certainly acceptable.

NOTE: A highly absorbable, gently effective form of vitamin C is *calcium ascorbate* (the form used in the BioSlim Formulas).

Vitamin D

This fat soluble vitamin must be taken in moderation to avoid possible overaccumulation in the body. Vitamin D is used in the absorption and utilization of calcium in the body. Recent research indicates that vitamin D may also help prevent certain forms of cancer (breast, colon). Obese people tend to have lower levels of this vitamin than non-obese individuals.

Vitamin D is found in certain fish, eggs and organ meats. It is also formed naturally in the skin when exposed to sunlight.

A reasonable dose of Vitamin D is 400 I.U. per day, though 800 I.U. is considered perfectly safe.

Vitamin E

This fat soluble vitamin is important in the body as a protector against chemical breakdown; it is therefore known as an *antioxidant* (as are vitamin C and selenium). Vitamin E is vital to cellular metabolism and oxygen utilization by the body. It also acts as a natural "blood thinner", helping to keep the circulation running smoothly. It strongly appears to help prevent heart disease *and* cancer.

Vitamin E is found in raw nuts, seeds, soybeans and especially in untreated wheat germ. A reasonable daily dose is 100 to 400 I.U., though 800 to 1200 I.U. is considered perfectly safe.

Vitamin K

Vitamin K, another fat soluble vitamin, is vital to blood clotting. It is also used in the utilization and storage of carbohydrates in the body, and is believed to be involved in several body functions vital to a long and healthy life.

Vitamin K is generally produced in the body by the friendly bacteria present in normal intestines; it is therefore not considered "essential" to ingest this fat soluble vitamin in the diet. Food sources include most green plants. A reasonable daily dose would be 40 to 70 mcg.

Bioflavonoids

Though not considered true vitamins, these substances function together with vitamin C in the body. They are important in the formation and strengthening of certain body tissues, particularly the body's smallest blood vessels, known as *capillaries.*

The best sources for bioflavonoids are fruits. There is no recommended dosage, though a combined dosage of all bioflavonoids of 75-100 mg per day is advised.

MINERALS

Minerals are inorganic elements, like *calcium, iron* and *zinc,* that are used in the body as vital parts of living tissue. They are mostly linked with enzyme complexes, serving many essential chemical roles in the body's daily functions. There is much cooperation between vitamins and minerals. Often they are intimately related both in function and absorbability in the body.

There are two broad types of minerals: "macro-minerals" present in large amounts in the body (e.g., calcium, magnesium, potassium and sodium) and "trace minerals", such as zinc, chromium and iron. All are vital to good health.

The following is a list of the most important minerals, appropriate-and-safe daily dosages, and basic functions. Keep in mind that the macrominerals calcium and magnesium are, in a balanced diet, typically ingested in sufficient amounts so that supplementation need not be the full daily requirement. Finally, note that certain minerals are in such plentiful supply that they are not addressed here, including phosphorus, sulfur, chlorine, and to a large extent, though not always, potassium.

THE ESSENTIAL MINERALS (with safe dosage ranges)

| Calcium | 300 – 1200mg | Part of all bones & teeth. Heart and nerve function. Blood clotting. Important partner in body with magnesium. |
| Magnesium | 300 - 800 mg | Extremely important, often deficient. Found mostly inside cells. Vital to food metabolism, nerve function, heart function, muscle action, energy utilization, blood sugar metabolism, hormone function, prevention of kidney stones, handling of fat, etc. |

Chromium	50 - 800 mcg	Vital to sugar and fat metabolism, and insulin function. Commonly deficient. May help control food cravings. Best form = polynicotinate.
Copper	1 - 3 mg	Hemoglobin/red cell formation. Body tissue maintenance. Protein metabolism. Nerve function.
Iodine	100 - 150mcg	Part of thyroid hormone, vital to all body functions & metabolism.
Iron	10 - 18 mg	Present in every cell of the body. Part of hemoglobin in red cells. Protein metabolism. Energy maintenance & oxygen delivery to body cells.
Manganese	2 - 10 mg	Important adjunct to several vitamins. Food metabolism. Nerve function. Thyroid function. Cholesterol metabolism.
Molybdenum	50 - 300 mcg	Used in iron metabolism. Important to the handling of fats in the body.
Selenium	50 - 300 mcg	Natural antioxidant. Preserves tissue elasticity. Hormone function. May prevent heart disease.
Zinc	10 - 30 mg	Vital and ubiquitous in the body. Aids in digestion and various aspects of metabolism, including energy production, healing, sex organ function, and sugar metabolism (it is part of insulin). Found reduced in obesity.

Finally, the mineral *Silicon*, not mentioned above, is thought to be important in the maintenance of the body's connective tissues, such as bones, tendons, cartilage and blood vessels. It is supplied in organic form in plant-derived, high fiber foods, and in some high quality formulations in the form of the herb *Horsetail*. All the above minerals are in the BioSlim Formulas.

OTHER NUTRIENTS

Essential Fatty Acids (EFAs), (see also above) can be provided to the body in the form of unsaturated fatty acids from unprocessed food, or in the more absorbable, more usable forms of GLA, EPA and DHA (*docosahexaenoic acid*)—often collectively as simply "the EFAs". (Note: GLA is an *Omega-6* fatty acid, while EPA and DHA are categorized as *Omega-3* fatty acids.)

The EFAs are important to many body functions, including: hormone formation; thyroid and adrenal gland functions; oxygen utilization; and a variety of other cellular functions. They have also been found helpful in the treatment of obesity.

Other nutrients, such as **CoQ10** (Coenzyme Q10), **SOD** (SuperOxide Dismutase), the bioflavonoid **quercetin**, and many others are not yet fully understood. They do not have the status of vitamins. Yet each is being studied with great interest around the world for its beneficial effects on the human body. In time, with more information, they may be assigned specific dosages. For now, they are used as for specific purposes only, by those familiar with their effects on the body.

Of particular interest is CoQ10, on which much research has been done in Japan and Europe. It appears to be beneficial in many ways, such as in relation to the heart. One of its benefits appears to be its ability to help in weight loss.

DANGEROUS PRODUCTS

Not everything that is "natural" or found in a health store is safe. In the area of dieting, there are certain nutritional supplements being marketed today that are potentially quite dangerous; specifically, these are the ones using the herb *ephedra,* also known as *ma-huang,* often in combination with *caffeine,* sometimes in combination with both caffeine and *aspirin* or the herb *white willow bark,* which contains aspirin compounds.

Ephedra is a naturally occurring stimulant that can actually help in weight loss. But its effect is a *chemical stimulation* of the body. The same is true of caffeine, though to a somewhat lesser extent. The problems here are many:

1) Ephedra can cause cardiac arrhythmias (irregular heart rhythms).
2) Both caffeine and ephedra work only as long as they are ingested, with no significant long-term benefits. They are quite drug-like in their effects. As soon as the dosages are stopped, the effects are lost. Which means you would have to continue taking these drug-like substances *forever* in order to maintain their effect. Taking *natural* supplementation, on the other hand, helps your body change *permanently*, by providing the body what it needs to change for the better, *not* by exerting a temporary chemical effect on it.
3) When these products are stopped, a "rebound" phenomenon may occur. Your weight can come back, with a vengeance.
4) Aspirin can cause stomach ulcers.
5) Excessive caffeine intake may cause headaches, heart irregularities, and may contribute to ulcer formation.

For these reasons the use of ephedra, aspirin and caffeine-containing supplements is specifically opposed.

Other so-called "supplements" to avoid include those "fat-burning pills" that pop up from time to time. These may or may not be dangerous, but they are certainly mostly useless.

In general, look at the ingredient list of any packaged item you put in your mouth. And look at the source. The maker of a food supplement should be a reputable company, with qualified experts—doctors, preferably—doing the formulations.

F O U R T E E N

THE BIOSLIM FORMULAS
ርጓ៩०

Most people who have experienced the BioSlim system report that the *Vita/Min Plus* and *SlimTone Formula* products were central to their success. These formulas contain every nutrient the body needs to metabolize food, normalize weight, and provide you with the sense of good health and well-being you want. Descriptions of most of the ingredients in these formulas may be found in the preceding chapter. In addition, SlimTone Formula has a special, proprietary herbal blend designed specifically for BioSlim for maximum effect.

The purpose of these nutrient formulas is to improve the nutritional status of the body so as to maximally aid in the achievement of weight loss and excellent health. These are not drugs! They are powerful, highly effective, all-natural formulas designed to provide your body virtually everything it requires.

They do not have to be taken forever. Once you have achieved your goals of good health and weight normalization, you may choose to taper down or stop one or both of the formulas. It is recommended, though, that a good multi-vitamin be taken routinely, if not Vita/Min Plus. Many people find they feel best when taking some amount of SlimTone on most days— typically from one to four tablets. These decisions will be yours; they should be based on your body's signals and needs.

The BioSlim Formulas are made of the finest, most absorbable, most beneficial ingredients possible. They are the best of the best. Many products on the market today use cheap, ineffective ingredients, so that taking them is quite futile. The

BioSlim philosophy is to use the best available formulations and get maximum results *now*.

Note that, in general, there are no known contraindications to taking the BioSlim Formulas. (However, if you suffer from severe heart disease, or any serious illness, or if you are pregnant, consult your physician. And read the appropriate section(s) under *Medical Considerations* above.)

The following is a description of how the BioSlim Formulas are used, and what effects to look for.

SLIMTONE FORMULA

To best gauge your individual reactions and needs, **BEGIN WITH TWO TABLETS 2–3 TIMES PER DAY with plenty of water**, *without* food if possible. Increase this dose as described below. Most people find that they do best with two tablets 3 times per day (total of 6 tabs per day), or even 2 tabs 2 times per day (total of 4 tabs per day). Some need as many as 3 tabs 3 times per day.

Four tablets at a time is also possible, but usually only once or twice per day; only a small percentage of people find this necessary. On the other side of the spectrum are those who use only one tab at a time, only two or three times per day. **It is vital to gauge your own reactions and adjust the dosage accordingly.** You know you're taking too much if you're experiencing such symptoms as too much energy, or too drastic a change in your bowel habits. These manifestations are often transient, lasting only a few days. Some people find that it takes some time to get the body used to the abundance of nutrients present in these formulas. See the *Solving Problems* chapter below for more information on what to do if you experience any unexpected reactions or changes.

You should increase your dose if you feel a lack of energy, or if your appetite or weight do not change despite following all other aspects of the program. Again, see the *Solving Problems* chapter below for more information.

Always take SlimTone tabs with plenty of water (1 cup is sufficient). While best taken *without* food, if you forget to take them until after you've started or finished eating, you should take them anyway. **The *best* time to take SlimTone Formula is 20-30 minutes *before* meals.** This is to maximize its absorption and effect on appetite, *not* because it's more effective if followed by a meal. In fact, you may take SlimTone *anytime between meals*.

Try to take SlimTone three separate times during the day, but settle for two separate times.

AFTER YOU REACH YOUR WEIGHT GOAL, you can cut down on your dosing of SlimTone. For maintenance, many people find that 2 or 3 tabs per day, all in the morning, works very well. Some find that they want to continue their SlimTone Formula as before, while others find they no longer need it at all, once they *feel good* and have *reached their target weights*. Experiment to see what works best for you.

VITA/MIN PLUS

This is the highest quality, most effective multi-vitamin-mineral formula you're ever likely to find. If you've been taking any kind of other multi-vitamin—STOP! (Note: calcium, magnesium, vitamins C or E, and EFAs are OK to add, if you wish.)

Normal dosing is 6 tabs per day, in two or three doses during the day, **ALWAYS WITH FOOD**. If you experience stomach upset, first make sure you're taking your tabs with sufficient food, and if you are, *reduce* your dose to 1 tab at a time until your body gets used to this potent multinutrient.

Some people find that 3 or 4 tabs per day is best for them, but usually, 2 tablets taken with each of three meals (or snacks) or 3 tablets taken with each of two meals works quite well.

Note that a yellowing of the urine is perfectly normal; it is caused by the B-vitamins (especially B-2) in Vita/Min Plus.

The criteria to determine how much to take are similar to the ones used for SlimTone Formula.

DO NOT TRY TAKING VITA/MIN PLUS WITHOUT AT LEAST SOME FOOD! At least a snack. Reason: These tablets are designed to be highly *absorbable* and *effective*. Taken without food, they can absorb so rapidly and so well that you may experience some stomach discomfort. Also, the vitamin *niacin* (vitamin B3) in these tabs—often used in large doses to help reduce cholesterol levels—can cause a temporary (15-20 minute) *flushing* of the skin which can be both unexpected and uncomfortable, if the tabs are taken on an empty stomach. This reaction is perfectly benign and normal and happens to almost *everyone* who takes niacin in sufficient quantity. If you take 2-3 tablets at a time WITH FOOD, this should not happen to you.

AFTER YOU REACH YOUR WEIGHT GOAL, you may choose to cut down on your dosing of Vita/Min Plus. Since this formula is also an excellent all-around multi-vitamin-mineral, though, many people choose to continue with it. Others find that, for maintenance, 2–4 tabs per day all in the morning or split into two doses works very well, ***always with food.***

As with SlimTone, you can and should experiment to see what works best. Ultimately, *you* decide what is best for you.

WHAT EFFECT?

What effect will these Formulas, combined with the BioSlim System, have on you? Answer: it's different for every individual. You, for example, may feel wonderfully improved. Your friend may feel only small changes. Everyone is unique, with a unique biochemical makeup. If, for example, you have a thyroid deficiency you don't know about, you may feel *better* on the BioSlim system, but not completely so until your condition is treated by a physician. If, on the other hand, you have significant nutritional deficiencies of which you are unaware (and it's very difficult to know this without extensive analysis), you are likely to benefit dramatically from the BioSlim system.

In short, there is no way to know in advance how ***dramatic*** your improvements will be, but we know that ***you can***

significantly improve your health and sense of well-being with the BioSlim System. There is no question about that.

Many people want to know what, if any, side effects they may experience with BioSlim. The fact is that most people do not experience side effects so much as *side benefits,* defined as benefits and improvements that were not expected. This occurs because as the body becomes healthier, *it fixes itself.* The BioSlim System is designed to give your body the tools it needs to accomplish this. The process itself is completely natural, and stems from the body's innate healing abilities. In fact, weight loss is itself a natural consequence of this process.

Other effects you may experience when first starting BioSlim: Vita/Min Plus will cause urinary yellowing (from the B-vitamins), and may upset your stomach if taken without food. Either Formula may increase energy levels to undesirable heights, though this is easily remedied. You may experience a change in bowel habits or a change in urinary patterns. You may initially even experience a slight headache until your body adjusts to its new, healthier internal condition.

Most people feel wonderful from day one. But with the intensive change for the better that BioSlim brings, the body can undergo some dramatic changes, including the removal of accumulated toxins and waste. This *detoxification* process can itself cause some transient symptoms. All these effects are generally temporary: they pass in a few days. You may wish to reduce the dose of one or both of the Formulas (see above) then wait to see how your body reacts before adjusting your doses to optimal levels. Use how you *feel* as a guide.

If you have specific questions or reactions about which you would like more information, e.g., if you weight loss is too slow or too fast, please refer to the *Solving Problems* chapter below. And remember to follow all instructions carefully, particularly the ones concerning *when* and *with what* to take the Formulas.

And have patience. You are in a *process*; it can take some time. It took your whole life to get to where you are today—it is reasonable to expect that it may take a few weeks or more to really change things.

OPTIONAL: ADDING NUTRIENTS

The BioSlim program is quite complete. Most people do not need to add anything to the plan. Additional supplementation is optional, though some may be needed for specific purposes.

Here are some nutrients that can be added to BioSlim:

- **CALCIUM AND MAGNESIUM:** These two minerals should always be taken in balance, preferably not more than 3 parts calcium to 2 parts magnesium. You may wish to add an extra 500–750 mg of calcium and up to 500 mg more of magnesium, particularly if you are a woman approaching or past menopause. The calcium and magnesium in the BioSlim Formulas are provided in highly absorbable forms, so that the amounts provided, combined with the BioSlim Food Plan, should provide most people with all they need.

- **ESSENTIAL FATTY ACIDS** (EFAs): Essential vitamin-like substances, these are necessary to proper hormone function and body tissue health. If you suffer from dry skin, weak nails, or menstrual difficulties you may need some extra EFAs. (See above or index for more details.)

- **SPIRULINA:** This is not actually a nutritional supplement, but a powdered, natural, extraordinarily healthful food. It is effectively fat-free, and loaded with protein, vitamins, minerals, and beta carotene. It does, however, taste awful. Instructions on the use of spirulina can be found in the *BioSlim Food Plan* chapter above (*Spirulina for breakfast?*).

- **LACTOBACILLUS:** See above or index for details. In short, these are the friendly, beneficial intestinal bacteria that help your body digest food and create certain vitamins. After treatment with antibiotics or any illness, the balance of these bacteria can be severely altered in the body. It is then very helpful to rebalance your system by taking lactobacillus supplements. They are particularly helpful for women who suffer from chronic or recurrent yeast infections. Gargling and swallowing this powder with water may be helpful in cases of sore throat.

- **MISCELLANEOUS**: Extra vitamin C may be taken, if desired, and some choose to take extra vitamin E (see previous chapter). Digestive enzymes (besides the bromelain in the formulas) may be utilized if desired and needed.

In general, exercise good judgment. Do not overdo anything. Keep all supplementation to levels consistent with that which nature intended for the human body.

FIFTEEN

THE ACTIVITY PLAN

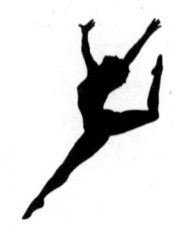

The credit belongs to the one who is actually in the arena, whose face is marred by dust and sweat; ...who strives valiantly... who knows the great enthusiasms, the great devotions...

Theodore Roosevelt

The importance of proper physical activity cannot be overemphasized. Properly done, it is one of the most beneficial positive actions you can take to support, strengthen, and rejuvenate your body.

As you lose weight, your body burns fat for energy, but it can also eat up muscle tissue—making you weaker, and *less able to lose weight*, a phenomenon familiar to many chronic dieters who always seem to find the beginning of each new diet program far more rewarding in terms of weight loss than subsequent phases. This occurs at least partly because muscles are very avid users of energy (i.e., calories) in the body, and if there is less muscle mass present to use up excess available energy (calories), clearly there will be less energy used. It's as if you're burning fuel and 30% of your furnaces shut down: the result is less fuel—in our case, calories—used up per day. As the rate at which you burn calories (your *metabolic rate*) diminishes, so does your rate of weight loss, and your ability to control your weight.

This is why dieting is such a difficult proposition, and why so many dieters fail to achieve their goals permanently.

The answer to this dilemma lies in taking great care when attempting to lose weight: it must be done right. That means, first of all: NO DIETING!—the primary principle of BioSlim. It also means eating the right foods *permanently*, and making sure you get the right nutrients into your body so that it can function correctly and *normalize* itself naturally. And, unquestionably, the answer must include a program of *reasonably sufficient* physical activity. You don't have to go out and buy every exercise video tape on the market today—or any at all, for that matter. You don't even have to go to the gym, or put on shorts. But you *do* have to get active! Even if it's just increasing your daily routine of walking, gardening, swimming or game-playing. When you do this, you'll be able to lose mostly *fat* instead of muscle. In fact, if you're determined, you can *increase* your lean body/muscle mass during the weight losing period, which can make losing fat *easier* as time passes.

In the companion *BioSlim Activity Plan* book, there are described many ways to achieve a level of physical activity that is right for you—ways that will, together with the rest of the BioSlim program, assure your *permanent* success.

You will be happy to note, too, that the benefits of regular, energetic physical activity don't stop with weight loss. They extend to many important aspects of your life. For details on the following list of improvements, see your *Activity Plan* book:

- Cardiovascular Health
- Bone Density And Bone Longevity
- Energy Levels
- Digestion And Bowel Function
- Reduction Or Elimination Of Depression
- Improvement of Muscle Tension and of Many Musculo-Skeletal Pain Syndromes
- Promotion of Good Blood Circulation
- Longevity — yes, you can live longer!
- ...and many more.

To realize all these benefits, it is *not* necessary to study and follow long, esoteric lists of exercises, or to tie yourself to a video cassette player, or even go to regular exercise classes. While each of these can certainly help—and for those who are able and wish to do so they can be very beneficial—they are not essential. As detailed in the *Activity Plan* book, you can gain the many benefits of proper physical activity by performing such simple everyday activities as walking, climbing stairs, swimming, bicycling, or even sitting or stepping up and down. Studies indicate that most of the advantages gained by exercise can be accrued with surprisingly mild, common activities—if they are done correctly and in sufficient quantities.

Also, you are less likely to injure yourself walking or climbing stairs than you are, say, weight-lifting or starting an aerobics class for which you are not well prepared.

Whichever direction you decide to take — get active! And remember the most important rule of exercise/activity: always *stretch* appropriately and always warm up and warm down. See the companion *Activity Plan* book for many more details on the importance and methods of proper stretching.

DIET AND ACTIVITY

Generally, following the BioSlim Food Plan and taking the Formulas (see earlier chapter) is all you need do about your nutrition. A new activity program, however, does require some special attention to diet. The points to remember are:

- NEVER EAT JUST BEFORE EXERCISING. The best time to get active is at least two hours after your last significant meal. Exercise diverts blood from the gastrointestinal tract to the muscles, and vice versa. For your body to efficiently digest and absorb a recent meal, it must have a sufficient blood supply to the stomach and intestines. Conversely, your muscles cannot function properly if some of the blood they require for proper oxygenation and nutritive support is busy in your intestinal area helping in the digestive process.

- AVOID HEAVY or LARGE MEALS BEFORE and AFTER EXERCISE. If you've just had a big, heavy meal, the two hour minimum mentioned above should be extended. Some meals take *all day* to digest! (Hopefully, you won't be eating too many of those on the BioSlim program.) This can once again lead to competition for blood supply between your body's muscles and your internal digestive organs.
- DRINK PLENTY OF FLUIDS before and after exercising. Whether you sweat profusely or not—whether you know it or not—you, like most people, probably lose more fluids than you realize during activity. Be sure to have lots of clean, pure water (*not* typically available from your faucet, but rather as bottled or "mineral" water) on hand. And be generous with yourself—drink heartily!

Unless you're body-building, these few pointers are all you need to know about how your diet interacts with your exercise program. (Note that body-builders require more calories and higher amounts of protein per day than other individuals.)

BASIC ACTIVITY PLAN TIPS:

For much more information, refer to the companion book, *BioSlim Activity Plan*.

- **START SLOWLY!** If you're "out of shape", take it easy! Build slowly, to prevent injury to your muscles, tendons, ligaments, and cardiovascular system. Injury is far more likely to occur to the unprepared. And an injury can truly cripple your efforts to achieve *all* your goals.
- **ALWAYS DO YOUR STRETCHES AND WARMINGS**: The most important part of any activity plan is stretching, which can be the *majority* of your plan. Follow the guidelines in the *Activity Plan* book.
- **CREATE AN ACTIVITY PLAN THAT'S RIGHT FOR YOU**: Do not feel obliged to follow *any* predefined activity plan. It is

perfectly acceptable, in fact, to avoid all structured exercises in favor of simply increasing your activity level with everyday lifestyle activities, such as walking up stairs instead of taking the elevator, walking or bicycling to the store instead of taking the car, swimming, gardening or going for long walks. You can find a hundred different ways to increase your level of activity without interfering with the way you lead your life. Do it!

- **ACTIVITIES DONE TO MUSIC** tend to be done longer and harder. Way it is.
- **CHECK WITH YOUR DOCTOR**: Before starting any exercise or any program of increased activity, you should tell your doctor, particularly if you suffer from any heart or lung ailment, or are under medical care for anything.

Remember that increasing your activity level is the single best way to increase your metabolic rate, so that you burn fat more efficiently and *faster*, not only while you're performing your activity, but *all the time*. When your metabolic rate goes up through regular physical activity, it tends to stay up, just like when it's down—as occurs with repeated unhealthful dieting—it tends to stay down.

Your Activity Plan, together with the entire BioSlim program, can become an irresistible force compelling you to achieve a leaner, healthier body.

SIXTEEN

THE SECRET POWER INSIDE YOU
ᎶᏋᎣ

All things are difficult before they are easy.
John Norley

R ead this chapter to yourself, aloud if you like, whenever your motivation feels like it's slipping. (Note: this chapter was written in consultation with Marc Bachrach, the noted California therapist and motivational expert.

Congratulations!

You've reaffirmed your decision to succeed! You've taken action!

OK, now take a moment to *congratulate* yourself. Congratulate yourself for using these words to motivate yourself. Using them to inspire yourself. To direct, to redirect, and encourage yourself to take deliberate action and to achieve the permanent success you truly desire. And you deserve ongoing, fulfilling success! So lets hear it for you! You have every right to cheer yourself on.

Redirect your mind and your actions toward one of your most desired... one of your deepest and most intensely wanted goals: To live, breathe, walk and enjoy a **TRIM, FIRM, HEALTHY AND ATTRACTIVE BODY.**

So go ahead: right now! Give yourself a pat on the back. You have taken action! And each action that you take leads to another.. and another.. and ANOTHER successful action. And soon you're in the grip of a positive habit.. a strong and healthy compulsion to eat the foods that make you TRIM, FIRM, HEALTHY

AND ATTRACTIVE, to enjoy the physical activity that nourishes your body with strength and vitality, and to use the BioSlim Formulas as directed and achieve complete success!

Yes. A POSITIVE habit! Positively desiring the right foods, thinking the right thoughts, taking consistent and successful action. Minute by minute, day-by-day you are creating a TRIM, FIRM, HEALTHY AND ATTRACTIVE BODY.

Consider this carefully: You have the right to a TRIM, FIRM, HEALTHY AND ATTRACTIVE BODY. You have the power to create it. No *thing* and no *one* has the right to take this opportunity away from you.

Now remind yourself: You don't *have* to lose weight. No one can *make* you lose weight or force you to. You know, just as certainly, you don't HAVE to stay heavy either. You have the RIGHT to make a choice. To choose right here.. and right now.. to live in a TRIM, FIRM, HEALTHY AND *RADIANTLY* ATTRACTIVE BODY. You have this right. You have the power to exercise this right. You have the desire and the necessary decision-making power to make it so. You're going to use these words to remind yourself over and over that you have the will to achieve and maintain the TRIM, FIRM, HEALTHY AND ATTRACTIVE BODY that you deserve.

You see, the WILL is not a function of grunting or groaning, or forcing... the will is a simple choice of *focusing* your mind on what you want. Repeatedly placing your attention on your desired goal: a TRIM, FIRM, HEALTHY AND ATTRACTIVE BODY. And when you focus your attention on creating the TRIM, FIRM, HEALTHY AND ATTRACTIVE BODY you deserve, when you focus cleanly, clearly, and powerfully on what you want, on what you deserve, on what will give you pride and satisfaction—then all of your thoughts, your emotions, your actions will get right into line, as focused and strong as a laser beam locked onto its target.

So let's line up now... Mind.. Body.. and Feelings. Imagine right here and right now what it's like to be in the TRIM, FIRM, HEALTHY AND ATTRACTIVE BODY that you desire and deserve. Take a few moments now to Mentally, Physically and Emotionally Imagine... Feel.. and Practice what it's like to be *walking*... in a TRIM, FIRM, HEALTHY AND ATTRACTIVE BODY... to be wearing the clothes that you'd so much like to be seen in. *Enjoy* looking good! Now remember: Your body is your billboard. It's the first thing that people see, and notice about you. Many people do make judgments on that basis alone. So it's in your best interest to advertise yourself as well as you possibly can.

And you *do* have the power to eat the foods that make you grow TRIM, FIRM, and most of all, HEALTHY. You know, you're not just making a body change... you're making a LIFE change, which is why you'll succeed completely and permanently. You have the Power to follow through with healthy, positive habit patterns. Powerful, Positive Habits. Almost as natural as breathing. Just like eating clean, healthy foods. Just like staying physically active, and following the BioSlim program. Just like all of these habits are becoming effortless and automatic patterns RIGHT NOW!

With each repetition, each positive thought and feeling, these positive, life-affirming addictions are anchoring themselves deeper and deeper into the habit-forming, behavior-producing, automatically functioning part of your mind. The same part of your mind that you trust every day to beat your heart and breathe when you're asleep. It knows what to do and how to do it! It IS learning. It IS absorbing. It IS responding positively to these ideas and your *actions*!

It's easy for you to create.. and *sustain*.. habits.. for habits are the job of your subconscious mind. With practice... with spaced repetition... the subconscious mind is *eager* and prepared.. to take on the habits that generate the most pleasure and the most satisfaction. There's nothing you have to do to *deserve* this power or these powerful habits—so just forget about past guilts, doubts, and worries about yourself. Instead, recognize that RIGHT NOW is your moment of power. You're beginning to realize now that you can experience the most pleasure when your energy level is strong and continuous. A

160 ♦ *The BioSlim Principles*

powerful level of vitality and wellness surging through your body makes you feel good!

So does the feeling of movement and "aliveness" when you enjoy performing your favorite physical activities. You realize now that the most difficult part of exercise is not the doing of it, but the <u>deciding</u> to be active—the *getting ready to do*.

And enjoy the activities you decide to do. Once you've actually begun, you know from past experience that it's easy to sustain and actually enjoy it! Just 30 seconds is all you need.. 30 seconds to begin the activity you know generates so much benefit and satisfaction. YOU HAVE THE RIGHT TO THESE 30 SECONDS! Focus now on how easy it is to do 30 seconds of physical activity. And then.. just keep going! You've already done the hardest part... STARTING! So just go ahead and finish! YOU HAVE THE RIGHT TO THESE 30 SECONDS! NO stress.. no external force has the right to take them from you.

You have the right to feel good. You have the power to take the next step forward... and the next... and the next! Hopelessness, helplessness, resignation, and rationalization... you simply refuse to buy into those old tired ways of feeling and thinking. You've released them now, along with the unnecessary unconscious patterns that you never chose on purpose, anyway! You're no longer a puppet of your ancient history.. no longer run by silly, thoughtless childhood commands to clean your plate or guilty pleas about starving children in other countries.

You're not going to play the role of garbage disposal at every meal—you're taking pride in pushing your plate away the moment you recognize you're not hungry! Your positive habits grow stronger and stronger each and every day. Since you have the right to enjoy a TRIM, FIRM, HEALTHY AND ATTRACTIVE BODY, you also have the right to protect that body; protect it from foods which poison it... foods which do nothing for you but add layers of inertia and extra pounds. Your positive addictions for healthy food, for clean food, and for physical activity are massively overwhelming the old outmoded eating habits, those accidentally-learned patterns of behavior that you've chosen to replace.

You're very clear now that the old eating habits you established early in childhood were not the result of your conscious choice. They were simply an accident of environment. Now, with your knowledge, with desire for health, you can choose to make a new choice. You no longer need to feel guilty, or under pressure. Anger, Resentment, Blame... let them go! You have the chance to feel clean and healthy, becoming more attractive to yourself and more attractive to others each and every day.

Following the BioSlim program, you ARE BURNING FAT. Burning fat and melting off excess pounds. And you are *not* "on a diet". You are not in prison. Not deprived or neglected. You are free to make choices. You allow yourself to feel free. You're not in jail and no one's judging you. Don't beat up on yourself for an occasional slip. Instead, get right back on track and focus on your REAL desire: A TRIM, FIRM, HEALTHY AND ATTRACTIVE BODY.

As you continue creating health and vitality, you'll find you just can't eat as much as you used to. The realization of this fact will become a source of pleasure and even pride. "Just can't eat as much as I used to" will become a commonplace thought, and a frequent statement to others. And as you become lighter and more active, the quality of your sleep will improve and life will become richer and more vibrant.

Congratulations... on creating the TRIM, FIRM, HEALTHY AND ATTRACTIVE BODY you so deeply deserve. Enjoy following the BioSlim program.

It's simple. And it works.... for *you!*

SEVENTEEN

MASTERING MOTIVATION
ೞ

> *There's no thrill in easy sailing*
> *when the skies are clear and blue,*
> *there's no joy in merely doing things*
> *which any one can do.*
>
> *But there is some satisfaction*
> *that is mighty sweet to take,*
> *when you reach a destination that*
> *you thought you'd never make.*
>
>   Spirella

This chapter deals with the psychological/motivational aspects of weight control and how you deal with food. It was written in consultation with motivational expert Marc Bachrach. The next chapter, dealing with cravings, addresses physical aspects and their interactions with psychological ones.

The facts, insights and tips described here can be used by anyone searching for ways to *gain control* over his or her life. The reader is urged to review these chapters more than once; each reading can bring new understanding and awareness.

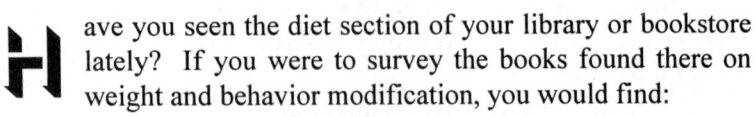

Have you seen the diet section of your library or bookstore lately? If you were to survey the books found there on weight and behavior modification, you would find:

- A huge number of reasons why people with weight problems eat the way they do;
- When and how they learned to reinforce these behaviors;

- Descriptions of the self image that goes along with this behavior pattern;
- The functions and payoffs that overeating and staying overweight provide.

You'd discover that the reasons and motivations for losing or gaining weight are minefields fraught with subtle traps and emotional quicksand. The reading is fascinating, filled with fact, theory, brilliant analyses and cogent insights—translated for the modern reader into the language, idioms, and style of the moment, beautifully arranged with life portraits and testimonial snapshots of "real people just like you".

Just a brief synopsis—even a brief *listing* of all these descriptions and theories—would fill the next 10 or 15 pages. Reading that list would take you on a thrilling, perhaps guilt-ridden odyssey into many possible variations of your past. Some individual books list more than forty or fifty different styles of overeating! One theory on the function of overeating actually links it to *ancestral memories in the subconscious mind*—memories of the time when we were cave people who needed to create body fat to survive cold weather and recurring famines!

OK. Maybe. Anything's possible...

But in truth, the reading is engrossing, and you would be amazed by all the mechanisms, rationalizations, and misconceptions most of us carry around as psychological baggage.

Rather than drown you in analytical detail on what you've already lived through and decided to change, let us instead offer a highly condensed version.

The bottom line.

All you *really* need to know about why, where, when and how you learned and reinforced your present habits, honed down to its true essentials, so that you may be free to take effective, immediate action, and *remain* successful.

WE ARE ALL OK

As a child, teenager, and young adult, you made the best decisions and choices you were capable of making, considering the input you were given. All of the reasons you learned to eat and carry weight the way you did make perfect sense on a number of levels and are *completely* reasonable and understandable.

You are not a criminal, not wrong, not a terrible person in any way. What you have done up to now worked... though it has generated its own share of pain and discomfort. It has made perfect sense up to the present moment.

You do not deserve eternal punishment, discipline, and internal criticism or nagging. Instead, you deserve compassion, support, and understanding *from* yourself *for* yourself.

You also deserve to make a new choice.

You can choose to live in a *slim, firm, healthy and attractive body*.

The same brilliant mechanism that learned, adapted, and produced the behaviors you now choose to release stands ready to serve as you input new choices and decisions into your new "bio-computer".

Start NOW, right here, where you are, with what you've got.

The Past is finished.

The Future isn't here yet.

Your Moment of Power is NOW.

Patience, self-love, persistence, realistic goals... These are your keys to a *slim, firm, healthy and attractive body*!

You know, last time we checked, being overweight a moral failing nor a serious character defect nor a sin nor an act harmful to others. Yet we've all been brainwashed with the "plain, hard truth" that the only proper corrective, the only effective approach, the only thing that should be used that has a prayer of getting results is harsh, authoritarian DISCIPLINE.

Nonsense! Actually, the truth is virtually the opposite. There are very few people indeed who can utilize a disciplinary, demanding style of "self-talk" to create behavioral change. Sooner or later, that famous (or infamous?) "inner child" in most of us will either rebel against or simply ignore the instructions entirely.

Most people respond most favorably, most easily, and most permanently to a kind, positive, and consistently supportive approach, especially when it is self-directed. This is a style of communication that is enthusiastic and direct, providing encouragement that conveys caring and real belief in our ability to succeed. Benevolent, concerned influence is the key, not punishment and control.

Apply the BioSlim Principles, then, and be kind to yourself. Flexing your spiritual muscles in this way may well yield benefits in areas you never thought to address.

A WAY TO EAT

Naturally thin people eat because they're genuinely hungry.

People with weight problems never really know what it's like to be hungry.

Naturally thin people, (people who have a *healthy* relationship with food) eat what they want. But when their bodies have had enough, they stop. They have an inner sense of what is *right* for their bodies. This decision is not an intellectual determination of how much food they "should" eat based on calorie counting or a food scale or what happens to be on a plate. It is an automatic habit triggered by real physical feelings in their bodies. If not hungry, they cannot be tempted, forced, or intimidated into eating.

People with eating problems eat because the food has an appealing taste or smell, because they might not have any for a while if they don't grab it now, or simply because it's there! They eat *mechanically,* using an automatic mechanism that turns itself on and off *independently* of their hunger. They can become gathering, shoveling, chewing, swallowing machines.

People with weight problems eat food to satisfy almost every possible kind of "hunger" (emotional "hunger", sexual "hunger", friendship "hunger", entertainment "hunger", etc.) *except the body's legitimate need for nutritious food.* The truth is, these "hungers" can never be fed by food! When food is used, it only serves to mask the underlying hungers temporarily and inadequately. When this happens, emotional truths are avoided, and the external or internal actions needed to deal with the *real* situation are thankfully delayed.

No matter how our language, our advertising media, or our role models try to convince us, the simple facts are: Food is *not* sex, food is *not* friendship, food is *not* entertainment, food is *not* comfort, food is *not* rest or relief from fatigue, and eating food does *not* meet the need to cry, laugh, shout, sing, or dance!

Those messages, as conveyed by all manner of enticing external, usually commercial signals, are typically presented in very clever, very effective ways. Their purpose is to program your mind to buy and consume the food being promoted — never to help you, never to get you to do the right thing for yourself.

When ingested in these confused and confusing ways, food can only serve as an unhealthy anesthetic, assaulting our bodies physically while doing nothing to help us deal with what we really need. Eating this way triggers an extra layer of guilt and anxiety (the "*vicious circle*" we'll deal with at the end of this chapter). Mechanically eating food for *any* reason other then legitimate hunger solves none of our problems, meets none of our real needs, and weighs us down physically, emotionally, and energetically.

SEPARATING REAL HUNGER FROM FALSE HUNGER

Infants and toddlers are completely in tune with their hunger. Have you ever tried to force an infant to swallow one morsel more than he or she needed as fuel? Chances are you ended up wearing it! At that point in development, there has been no corruption of the relationship between eating and the true needs of the body for fuel and food. That distortion doesn't happen until we're trained to associate food and eating behaviors as rewards, punishments, substitutions, and "important" events—behaviors we can "control" to gain recognition, approval, disapproval, and so on. With time, we learn to allow ideas, outside stimuli, and relationship struggles to distract us from and often *block* our awareness of our bodies' true hunger sensations.

Your major challenge in disconnecting yourself from unnecessary, habit-driven eating is separating out real hunger from false hunger.

First, the facts.

There are certain clues your body gives you when you are *truly* hungry, i.e., when your body needs food for its *physical* needs. Most commonly, it is that empty, "gnawing" feeling in the vicinity of the middle abdomen. It can also include feelings of mild lightheadedness, fatigue, or unexplained nervousness. Each of us has a different set of clues. Most of us know what they are. If you do not, there is a simple way to find out. Stop eating for 12 to 24 hours, drinking only water. Carefully watch your reactions, *listening* to your body until you clearly discern the true feeling of hunger.

Incredibly, many people have not felt true hunger for *decades*. If you are among them, do the simple, brief experiment just described, and <u>discover hunger</u>. Once felt, it will be easier for you to postpone eating until that same sensation is felt. And by the way, you're in for a treat. It can be *exhilarating* to feel true hunger when you haven't felt it in years. It makes you feel *alive*.

Beware of false urges to eat. These may be little more than muscle tensions triggered by some eating cue or cues, or psychological urges that have nothing to do with true, physical hunger. Those cues and urges can be "external" or "internal". Examples of external cues include seeing or smelling a particular food, the offer of food, or perhaps becoming aware of the time on the clock ("it's dinner time"). Internal cues and urges are often the emotional states (anxiety, frustration, boredom) and ideas about eating ("if I don't eat now, I'll be hungry later and may not be able to eat then.")

These muscle tensions and energetic or psychological sensations that you may feel in your body, and the thoughts and mental images that accompany them, are the most common sources of the urge to eat. But these urges, though frequently strong and compelling, are the markers of *false* hunger.

The areas of the mouth and throat deserve additional consideration. **THIRST** for liquid, not hunger for food, is what you really feel here. (See later in this chapter for more about thirst!) You may also feel the urge to bite and tear with the teeth, and the impulse to chew in the muscles of the jaw and mouth (and sometimes all the way through to the neck muscles). These occur without the presence of real hunger, but are instead often linked to emotional states, such as frustration, anger or depression. Sometimes, they arise from an urge to clean the mouth and throat. They are generally *not* signals of the body's need for energy-producing, life-sustaining fuel.

Each of us is motivated in many ways to eat. Much of that motivation has more to do with conditioning—or *habit*—than with real physiological need. Remember the Russian scientist Pavlov and his famous experiments with dogs? By associating the sound of a bell with the presence of food, he was able to *condition* the salivary response in a group of dogs he worked with. Soon, all he had to do was ring the bell, without the presence of food, and the dogs would salivate.

Instead of bells activating our nervous systems, we humans have words, images, restaurant signs, menus, TV, radio, friends, clocks, and hundreds of other cues. Just as Pavlov's dogs eventually did not need the presence of food to respond to the bell, so we humans often no longer need to be truly hungry in order to eat. We eat because some bell has rung.

One of the objectives of the BioSlim program is to return you to a full, permanent awareness of the food you ingest as fuel for your body. You want to use the cleanest, most efficient fuel available. And, naturally, the best-tasting and most aesthetically pleasing. Regarding the *amounts* of fuel you use: you would surely *never* fill up your car's gas tank and then unconsciously add another 10 gallons. You'd be standing in a dangerous fuming pool of gasoline if you did! Be similarly careful with your body.

Treat your body carefully. Use the same common sense principles you use in every other aspect of your life. Recognize the false urges and ignore them. Learn to identify *true* urges, like true hunger, and act on them. Don't overfill the tank. Don't explode.

TAKING ACTION

Here's a powerful aid to help you translate your newfound awareness into meaningful, satisfying *action*.

Let's establish a numerical scale to gauge your hunger for "fuel" (food) and stomach fullness. This 0-to-10 scale will assist you in becoming more conscious and more precisely aware of real hunger and healthy eating. (Remember: The goal is *eating only when hungry,* and then only as much as the body requires for fuel. The result is a *slim, firm, and attractive body!*)

THE HUNGER SCALE:

> 0— **TRUE STARVATION**, caused by lack of any food for several days. Abdominal discomfort, hunger pangs, weakness, fainting.
>
> 5— **NOT HUNGRY**. Neutral. Fueled but **NOT FULL!**
>
> 10– **BEYOND STUFFED**. Bloated and extremely uncomfortable physically. Completely turned off by even the idea of more food.

Decide to eat only when you're really hungry, and stop before you're completely full, after your hunger is satisfied. Try to never begin eating unless you are at 4 or below on the hunger scale. Practice checking your hunger level *by the numbers.* As you become more aware and more precise, you might make a game of not eating before you're at a 3!

170 ♦ *The BioSlim Principles*

Your target once you start eating is to stop when you reach 5, or even before. Not one *smidgen*, nor one *morsel* of food more! **You are choosing to regularly stop eating before you are full, but after your true hunger has completely disappeared—in total comfort and satisfaction.**

Each time you reinforce this vital, important habit, say to yourself, mentally or out loud: "I just can't eat as much as I used to." As your eating habits return to their natural normal state, this statement will become the absolute truth! *(Just for fun, hold up your hand and make a fist. This is about the size of your stomach! See now how much less food your body really needs?)*

If you experience any doubt or confusion, treat this feeling as NOT being hungry. Only a genuine, *physical* sensation can tell you when you are hungry. If you are in doubt — you are not!

- *Stop eating before you are "full"!*
- *Ask: "Am I hungry? What scale number am I at?"*
- *If you have to think about it, if there is any uncertainty, this is not hunger! It is a conditioned response, a behavior activated by a belief, a ritual, an external stimulus, or some other cue. It cannot be REAL hunger unless it is clearly felt. It is FALSE hunger!!*

There is some good news here. Just because your hunger-awareness faculty has been distorted, confused and left unused does not mean that it has been damaged or destroyed. Far from it! The simple process of *paying attention to your body's signals* and separating other surface sensations from it, *will* return to you your ability to be completely and consciously in tune with your internal signals for healthy, nutritious food.

You have the power to be in touch with the pure, unadulterated, unconditioned body sense of genuine hunger. Nothing and no one can remove it from your biological mechanism, not even you. The more you follow the BioSlim program and begin adopting its healthful eating style and nutritionally rich sources of fuel, the easier and more rapid will be your return to balance. Ultimately, you'll once again find the same clear, effective feedback system any child, animal, or naturally thin person uses to control the process of eating, without extra effort, confusion or discomfort. Patience, persistence, and a self-loving, attitude will carry you through to your goal.

Tell someone that one of the most important steps in the BioSlim system is to only eat when truly hungry, and they'll tell you how obvious that is. We should know—we've told LOTS of people! And guess what. The vast majority were unclear about when they were experiencing genuine hunger and how to recognize that feeling in their bodies!

Now close your eyes, breathe slowly and deeply a few times, place your awareness in your stomach (not your mouth, tongue, teeth, head, jaw, shoulders, back, eyes, or hands) and ask yourself: Am I hungry?

If the answer is "no", your body does not need or want food! Choose to turn your attention to whatever task is at hand or whatever enjoyment you might choose.

If the answer is "yes", decide if you want to eat right this moment or whether you may wish to eat later.

If you experience confusion or uncertainty when you ask these questions, YOU ARE NOT HUNGRY!! Choose to do anything else *except eating food!* With patience and repetition, you will become clearer and more in touch with *true* hunger.

No one is "always hungry". And there is no such thing as being "a little hungry"! Either your body needs and is requesting nutritious fuel, or it is not.

You deserve a simple, totally natural relationship to food as fuel and nutrition. Soon, by repeatedly asking the question "Am I hungry?", your answer will become obvious every time the question is asked. In time, you'll find it unnecessary to ask! Think of using this question in the same way you used training wheels when you were learning to ride a bicycle. Eventually, they came off and you rode without them.

Here are some powerful ways to assist yourself in staying conscious while you eat, and reorienting yourself to a more *natural* style of eating (defined as eating only when you're hungry, and only as much as your body needs for fuel, enjoying your food without guilt or drama):

1. Put your fork or spoon down after EACH bite, until you've finished what you're chewing and have swallowed it. If you're eating finger food or a sandwich, choose to put it down on your plate after each bite. The point is to remove as much of the automatic, unconscious, habit-based aspect of overeating as possible. Slowing down the eating process in this way will allow you to stay more aware of the responses arising in your mouth, taste buds, stomach, and the rest of your body, and will enhance your ability to achieve full control.

    If you find this at all uncomfortable, you may add a slow, deeper-than-normal breath between bites. The first time you do this, treat it as an experiment, allowing yourself time to find a way to make it easy and natural.

2. Look at the food on your plate before you begin eating. Become aware of its quantity. Roughly determine what HALF of this meal consists of. Decide in advance that when you reach this halfway point in your meal you're going to take a pause and STOP EATING COMPLETELY! (Make sure the half you choose is protein-carbohydrate balanced, per the *Food Plan*.)

    Halfway through, as you decided when you started, put your utensils and all food down on the plate, dish, or table. Breathe once or twice slowly, and turn your attention away from food as completely as possible. If you are eating with a companion, try asking a question and pay total attention to the answer and the ensuing conversation.

Or simply think about what you're going to be doing after the meal. Or you may wish to indulge in some daydream about anything that fascinates you.

After this eating interruption of *at least* thirty seconds, direct your attention to your stomach and decide what number on the hunger scale you're at. If you've reached a 5—if you're no longer hungry—push your plate away. You're finished!

3. Sometimes you may find it difficult or confusing to be clear about your hunger level while you're eating a meal. If you cannot tell whether you're hungry or not, **decide at that moment to finish just two more bites of food.** Choose the very best, most appealing, most appetizing bites on the plate or in the meal. This is the part of the meal you usually save to the very end because it's so enjoyable. This is the taste you want left in your mouth when the meal is over. (That's "when the meal is over", as opposed to "when all the food is completely gone".) Enjoy these last two scrumptious bites thoroughly!

Then—pause briefly, and ask your body again about where on the hunger scale it is. If you're still confused, or you get no signals at all, chances are you are no longer truly hungry for food as necessary body fuel. If you were to continue eating, you would be following outmoded rituals and concepts about eating, rather than truly feeding your body what it needs. Examples of such rituals and ideas: "I have to finish everything on my plate." "Take all you want but eat all you take." "If I don't eat all this now, I won't have anything until....o'clock." "I ate junk earlier so I have to eat every bit of this healthy food to balance it out." Etc., etc.

It is time to demonstrate your mastery over food! Choose to end your meal, strengthening your confidence in the process.

With practice, your awareness of the hunger signals in your stomach will grow more accurate and more definitive. Soon, being clear and immediately conscious of them will be an easy, natural part of your life. There will come a time when you will find it hard to believe you ever ate any other way!

4. As mentioned earlier, try writing down everything you decide to eat *before* you eat it, but *after* you decide you *want* to eat it. This action alone is highly effective in helping people control their eating and weight levels.

THIRST IS NOT HUNGER

"Am I thirsty?"

Acting on this simple question may be the most powerful thing you can do to reclaim your naturally healthy, lean body.

Try asking "Am I thirsty?" whenever you sense a message from your head or body that prompts you to crave food. If that message is "I want *something*" instead of "I need to eat", there is a very real possibility that your body craves *fluid,* not food.

When you feel the urge to eat, take a drink of water instead of eating food! Then ask yourself what number you're at on the hunger scale. Often you will find that the urge to eat is no longer there! This is because sometimes our minds learn to confuse any kind of "craving" as a need to eat food. Yet often our bodies are simply thirsty, because most of us don't drink as much water as our bodies need every day! Knowing this, and supplying your body with what it *truly* needs, can have a dramatic impact on your automatic-eating machinery, and on your self-confidence.

Simple question, simple answer, simple action.

"Am I thirsty?"

This kind of approach is the essence of the BioSlim method: Keep it simple; take it easy; make it work *for you.* The healthy, natural way.

Your allies are:
- Patience
- Acceptance

- Repetition

This is NOT about substitution. You're making sure you're getting what you need, when you need it, *because* you need it.

Congratulations! You *deserve* to get what you need.

NATURALLY THIN

Let's review again how naturally thin people eat.

They (and *you* in the near future!) consider only four things:
1) Whether they're hungry or not
2) Precisely what they want to eat
3) What they're putting in their mouths and its immediate effect on them
4) When their bodies have had enough food

That's all you really need to know and act upon to be released from automatic eating behavior—to be free to create a *slim, firm, healthy and attractive body*!

MENTAL TOOLS

There are some of the mental tools you can use anywhere, anytime to promote awareness and action, and to further help reestablish a natural, biologically sound, healthy relationship between your body and food. These tools can help change the nature of your mental questioning from <u>re</u>active to <u>pro</u>active, which can dramatically strengthen your movement into this healthy mind-set.

Examples of <u>re</u>active mental processes: "Why did I do that?" "How could I be so stupid?" "When am I ever going to get control?" The more effective, <u>pro</u>active approaches (those that deal with situations in advance), are described below.

Consider the following questions as your additional keys to unlocking the prison of unconscious, automatic behavior.

You can apply these questions anytime you have a thought about eating or an impulse to put something in your mouth. The more often you ask them, learn from them, think about them and act on the information they yield—the faster you'll dissolve the old automatic-eating machine and find your new, naturally healthy eating system.

1) Am I thirsty?
2) Am I hungry?
3) What number am I at on the 1-to-10 hunger scale?
4) What does my body want to eat?
5) Crunchy or soft?
6) Sweet or salty?
7) Spicy or mild?
8) Besides eating, what other options or activities are available to me?

Many people have discovered (after determining that they are *neither* truly hungry nor thirsty) that rather than ignore the impulse or "urge" to eat, they can *extinguish* the strength of the impulse rather than empowering it by fighting! The event then exhausts itself because it is no longer pushing against anything or in conflict with the "will". Your attitude is simply that you have been handed a message about something that no longer interests you. You thank the messenger in an easy-going, disinterested manner, then carry on with your life's business.

The mental dialogue might go something like this.

- I feel an urge to eat.
- I *could* eat if I choose to.
- I could eat, but I don't have to eat.
- I am the one who chooses.
- I've decided to eat food when I'm actually hungry.
- I notice a physical sensation in my (mouth, hands, face, jaw....wherever) and a thought in my mind about eating.
- *Wow*, is my....(mouth, face, jaw... wherever) tense!
- I have an urge to eat.

- But I am not this urge.
- I am the one who is aware of the urge.
- I am the one who chooses.
- The urge will pass, yet I remain—I, the one who is aware — I, the one who chooses.
- I choose to allow this "urge", this echo of the past, to diminish and end; to spend its energy and end its mission.
- It has reminded me of a choice.
- And I have chosen.
- I could eat if I choose to.
- I choose to eat when my body is actually hungry for nutrition and fuel.
- I am the one who chooses. I am the one who is aware. I am awake, alive, and actively choosing.
- I *choose* health.
- I *choose* freedom.
- I *choose* to separate real hunger from false hunger.
- I *choose* power and liberation, not slavery.

COURSE CORRECTIONS

The purpose of using the BioSlim system is the achievement of permanent, long lasting success. NOT immediate perfection and overnight euphoria.

Consider yourself a guided missile. You've set your target and plotted your course. Inside this missile is a guidance system that informs the missile's computer whenever the missile strays off its predetermined course. This makes it possible for the computer to make the course corrections necessary to reach its chosen target. It provides this essential, up-to-date information just as any efficient feedback system does. It does this without judgment or criticism. It DOESN'T flood the computer with waves of emotional overload, or play audio tapes of old reprimands from its parents over the loudspeakers at full volume. It DOESN'T blame the missile or demand that it instantly abandon the mission as hopeless. IT JUST HELPS CORRECT THE COURSE—by providing accurate, reliable information about where it is and what needs to happen to get back on course. It repeatedly and rapidly *learns* from "mistakes", gathering the facts necessary to correct its course and get back "on target".

The past is finished—over and done with! It is history. All that remains from the past are memories and learned responses. The future hasn't happened yet and must be created, with specific purpose, to the best of your power and intention. Just as the missile's guidance system takes information from the present and helps the missile reach its target in the future, so does your past exist only as a launching pad from which to accelerate in a clear and self-correcting manner into the future.

Your conscious awareness will tell you when you're off course, so you can effectively make the right course corrections.

Yes, you have the right to berate yourself, judge yourself harshly for any slip, and turn away from your eventual success because of momentary pain and aggravation. Consider, however, that YOU CREATE FOR YOURSELF much of that discomfort with the way you give yourself critical feedback. It may also be true that you might not treat anyone else in the world as harshly, as punitively, and with as little support and encouragement as you treat yourself in such moments. Are you harder on yourself than anyone else you interact with? You may have lots of "good reasons" why you MUST punish and overwhelm yourself with helplessness, guilt, suffering, and pain whenever you make a mistake. But are those reasons valid?

Now is the time to realize that *mis*-takes provide the only opportunities you have for the "*re*-takes" that ultimately create the success you desire and deserve!

THE VICIOUS CIRCLE AND HOW TO END IT

Recognize the following scenario? You overeat once and begin to flood yourself with discouragement. Your guilty feelings and self-critical thoughts generate anxiety and discomfort. A vicious circle is formed. Anxiety leads easily to more overeating, which then triggers further discouragement and guilt.

REFUSE TO BEGIN THE CIRCLE before it even starts by simply shrugging off your mistake with compassion and self-acceptance. A slip does not invalidate your previous progress! Recognize, then forget the all-or-nothing

> *"I-have-to-have-total-absolute-perfect-control-and-immediate-permanent-success-or-I'm-an-incompetent-miserable-doomed-failure"*

brand of thinking. Return to the relaxed, tension-free BioSlim method of creating a *trim, firm, healthy and attractive body.*

Remember, you *can* and you *will* lose your extra weight... easily and naturally... painlessly and permanently. Using BioSlim as a conscious commitment to yourself, you *choose* to no longer deprive yourself of a *trim, firm, healthy, and attractive body.*

You deserve it.

You owe it to yourself.

Enjoy it!

Eighteen

WHAT TO DO ABOUT THOSE CRAVINGS
☙❧

There are two broad categories of causes of cravings. The first is mostly psychological, having to do with triggering stimuli such as:

- "It's time to eat"
- A smell
- Some event or activity, like sitting in front of the TV
- Some place you find yourself in
- Some person
- Some feeling
- Etc.

This area has been covered at length in the preceding *Mastering Motivation* chapter. *(Note: eating in front of the TV is not a good idea at all. You will end up eating far more than your otherwise would, and far more than your body actually needs.)*

But for most people, cravings—and the uncontrolled, unnatural eating they cause—are not *only* psychological in origin. They are caused by a complex set of factors: physical and biochemical causes intertwined with mind-related issues. As with all things related to the human condition, this is not simple.

To control "uncontrollable" cravings, you must apply solutions to *both* factors causing them: the physical *and* the psychological. Your probability of failure or recidivism will otherwise remain high.

Psychological factors and their solutions have been discussed earlier (see the *Mastering Motivation* and *Secret Power Inside*

You chapters). What, then, are the factors contributing to the *physical* aspects of cravings? Is there a chemical reason for your insatiable need to consume ice cream? Do those potato chips fill some kind of *physiological* need of which you are not aware?

WHY WE GET CRAVINGS, PHYSICALLY

The following are the most common types of physical disorders that can underlie the existence of cravings:
- Blood sugar disorders
- Thyroid dysfunction
- Depression
- Severe food allergies
- Nutritional deficiencies
- Food/Diet Imbalance

BLOOD SUGAR DISORDERS: A DISASTROUS CYCLE. See *Diabetes* in the *Medical Consideration* chapter above for more information on blood sugar. With regard to cravings, *hypo*glycemia, or *low* blood sugar (as opposed to the high blood sugar of diabetes) is usually the problem. Here's what happens: as blood sugar levels drop, certain symptoms occur: fatigue, lightheadedness, inability to concentrate, weakness, headaches, irritability, *and cravings*. The foods that are most often craved are those with the highest simple sugar contents: candies, cakes, cookies, ice cream, fruit juice, and sugar itself. But *any* food may be the object of the cravings that occur with hypoglycemia.

Hypoglycemia is itself often caused by poor eating. The eating of sweets naturally causes blood sugar to immediately rise. But often, within 60 minutes of this initial rise comes the beginning of the crash, as insulin floods the body moving sugar into your body's cells (and storing the excess *as fat*). Eventually, as the body responds to the high sugar levels caused by the high-sugar food with hormones (insulin) that *reduce* blood sugar, blood sugar levels often drop *below* the level that existed prior to the ingestion of the sweet food. This in turn creates a *craving* for more sweets (or fat), as the body calls out for *more food*, more sugar. And so the craving/binge cycle begins.

This cycle is exacerbated by caffeine, which acts as an additional, unnatural stimulant on top of the stimulation caused by the "sugar rush" created by the high-sugar food. So that doughnut and coffee you eat for breakfast (*not* under BioSlim, of course—right?) and again in mid-morning can be quite devastating to your whole day! It sets up a *whole day* of roller-coaster blood sugar levels, with each dip causing you to crave more sweets and/or more caffeine. This common syndrome causes irritability, mood swings, severe fatigue (particularly at the end of the day), headaches, and many other negative effects.

The solution: Break the cycle. *Stop* eating high-sugar foods. *Stop* eating all junk food. *Stop* eating white flour. Follow the BioSlim Food Plan. *Use* the BioSlim Formulas. And see *How to Prevent and Stop Cravings* below.

THYROID DYSFUNCTION: This disorder is discussed at length under *Thyroid Gland Disease* in the *Medical Considerations* chapter above, and below in the *Women: Special Facts and Considerations* chapter.

Thyroid deficiency, the most common thyroid disorder, causes a slowdown of most body functions. It can cause hypoglycemia (see BLOOD SUGAR DISORDERS immediately above), which in turn causes cravings. Thyroid deficiency may also cause excessive cravings directly, without invoking the mechanism of hypoglycemia.

The solution: Get your thyroid checked thoroughly (see the *Medical Considerations* chapter for test details). Get treatment if necessary. And see *How to Prevent and Stop Cravings* below.

DEPRESSION: The depressed individual often seeks solace in food (or, conversely, may in some cases shun food). Typically, the cravings experienced come at unusual times, such as in the middle of the night. (Don't worry. If you have night-time cravings it does *not* mean you're clinically depressed; there are many other reasons for cravings.) Depression can lead to indiscriminate eating, which in turn leads to more or exacerbated depression due to the nutritional deficiencies and imbalances caused by poor diet. Another negative cycle is thus created.

The solution: See your physician. Use the BioSlim Formulas! Follow the BioSlim System as closely as possible. Avoid all sweets, alcohol and food additives. And see *How to Prevent and Stop Cravings* below.

SEVERE FOOD ALLERGIES: See *Allergies and Substance Sensitivities* in the *Medical Considerations* chapter above for more information on food and other allergies.

Food allergies can cause cravings because *we often most crave those foods to which we are most allergic or sensitive.* The reasons for this phenomenon are unclear. But it can cause prolonged, chronic dysfunction, including migraine headaches, sinusitis, recurrent respiratory and ear infections, severe recurrent gastrointestinal disorders, arthritic syndromes, and many others. These symptoms can be perpetuated by the constant need to ingest more of the causative foods, i.e., cravings.

The solution: Avoid all suspected allergenic foods and substances. *Vary* the diet: try never to eat any food, particularly those you suspect are allergenic, more often than once every four days. This should help reduce the severity of food-induced allergic symptoms and cravings. Avoid all junk foods and sweets. And see *How to Prevent and Stop Cravings* below.

In most cases the primary issue has more to do with diet than disease, disorder, or deficiency. What often happens is that bad eating begets more bad eating. Which leads us to our last two categories of causes of cravings:

NUTRITIONAL DEFICIENCIES: People who are deficient in one or more essential nutrients may eat prodigious amounts of food because their bodies crave the missing nutrients, and are looking for those nutrients in ever-increasing amounts of food.

Unfortunately, the body cannot choose the food it eats without processing the order through the brain, where other impulses often lead the choosing mechanisms astray. The food the body actually receives, then, is often devoid of the very nutrients it craves. This sets up an endless cycle of cravings and binges.

The solution: Avoid all sweets and junk food. Follow the BioSlim program as closely as possible. Use the BioSlim Formulas! And see *How to Prevent and Stop Cravings* below.

FOOD/DIET IMBALANCE: A little-known fact is that certain foods tend to create certain cravings. Eating a high-sugar food may cause you to crave salt, so you follow it with some potato chips. Conversely, salt may lead to a sugar craving, which is why you may follow potato chips with a piece of cake or ice cream, or soda pop instead of water. Sugar can also increase craving for fat and vice versa, a useful point to remember when attempting to make sense of your eating habits. One may rightfully expect, then, that potato chips, which are high in both salt and fat, would lead to a very powerful craving for something sweet. Sound familiar?

Below is a table containing some common cross-reactions between foods that underlie this very common and powerful source of cravings: a *food/diet imbalance*. These examples are designed to reflect the *pattern* of food-induced cravings.

COMMON CROSS-REACTING FOODS:

FOOD EATEN	CRAVING CAUSED
Salty Food	Sugar/ Sweets
Sweet / Sugar	Salty Food
Fatty Food	Sugar/ Sweets
Sugar/ Sweets	Fatty Food
Alcohol	Salty Food
Salty Food	Alcohol

Beer	Fatty Food
Beer	Salty Food
Chocolate	Salty Food
Salty Food	Chocolate
Chocolate	Fatty Food
Fatty Food	Chocolate
Coffee	Salty Food
Coffee	Fatty Food
Fatty Food	Coffee
Undiluted Fruit Juice	Salty Food
Salty Food	Undiluted Fruit Juice
Red Meat	Sugar/Sweets
Fowl	Sugar/Sweets
Butter or Cheese	Sugar/Sweets
Meat of any kind	Alcohol
Many drugs	Salty or Fatty Food

Use this list to help you understand why you sometimes eat the way you do—why you feel compelled at times to consume certain foods. Understanding the source of your cravings will dramatically improve your ability to conquer them!

HOW TO PREVENT and STOP CRAVINGS

BREAK THE CYCLE! Of all the physical causes of cravings listed in this chapter, all but one (thyroid dysfunction) represent negative, self-perpetuating cycles, including: blood sugar abnormalities, nutritional deficiencies, food/diet imbalance, allergies and depression.

It is vital to break each of these cycles! *Stop* eating and drinking excessive sweets. *Stop* eating nutritionally empty, depressing junk food. *Avoid* all allergenic foods. And *break* the habit of eating one cross-reacting food after another. These negative food cycles can often be permanently changed in a matter of a few days. All that is needed is the will to do it.

The following are suggestions for accomplishing the *breakage* of these cycles:

- **Food quality:** This is the most important factor you can change in the area of negative food cycles. *Follow the BioSlim Food Plan as closely as possible!* Avoid all junk food. Avoid all foods that trigger cravings. Eat only *real, recognizable* food.

- **Avoid all added fats:** There are at least three compelling reasons now to avoid all added fats and oils, per the BioSlim System. In no particular order, they are:

1) They will make you fatter faster than anything else you can do or eat.

2) They increase your risk of heart disease and cancer, and will shorten your life.

3) They cause you to crave sweets, which in turn damages your health, increases fat levels, and make you crave more fat!

- **Avoid sugar and excess concentrated carbohydrates:** Refined white sugar (table sugar) is damaging to your health in many ways, and will

a) directly cause weight gain, and

b) cause cravings for fats that will further cause weight gain. White sugar is one of the *worst* foods you can eat, second in infamy only to added fats and oils.

Highly concentrated carbohydrate foods, e.g. white bread, have a similar effect, destroying protein-carbohydrate balance.

- **Drink plenty of water:** This is an easy, healthful way to help avoid cravings. Often, **a perceived craving for food, particularly fatty food, may be easily satisfied with a cup or two of water.** Drinking plenty of water also helps to naturally control appetite through a direct effect on the stomach. Always drink pure, fresh water; avoid tap water laden with chlorine and other chemicals.

- ***Try brushing your teeth instead of eating!*** Often, a craving for a particular food, especially high-fat, high-sugar food, is caused by something no more complicated than a bad taste in the mouth. A quick, refreshing tooth brushing or mouthwash rinse will often get rid of cravings immediately and painlessly. Or try using calorie-free mint drops, such as natural peppermint.

- ***Food timing:*** Do *not* skip breakfast; this only leads to hypoglycemia and severe cravings sometime around mid-morning, which in turn cause you to eat cookies or doughnuts with coffee and sugar, which in turn may set you up for a roller-coaster blood sugar ride for the rest of the day. *Not* a good idea.

   Avoid eating anytime within two or three hours of bedtime. Not eating anything near bedtime can change your eating patterns so that you are *hungrier* in the morning, leading you to indeed eat a decent-sized breakfast, which will then help control your mid-morning cravings.

   If you need to snack between meals, eat some fresh vegetables or some fruit, in moderation.

- ***Meal size:*** A pattern of smaller, more frequent meals throughout the day is much more conducive to craving control than a pattern of starvation or mild snacking during most of the day combined with one large (often *very* large) daily meal. Studies have also shown that spreading food intake throughout the day helps in the weight loss effort, while concentrating calories all in one large meal hinders it.

- ***Watch your salty foods***, if they lead to sugar cravings (or if you suffer from kidney disease or high blood pressure).

- ***Eat slowly:*** This will help minimize the effect of cravings, because you will find that you are satisfied *sooner* than you would be if you were wolfing your food down.

- ***Vary your diet:*** Useful when food allergies are suspected. Try to avoid eating any particular food, such as bread or other wheat product, eggs, meat, corn, soy, and any other potentially allergenic food too often. *Rotating* your diet, so that you do not consume any single allergenic food more often than *once every four days* is the easiest way to accomplish this.

- ***Read and follow*** the tips, ideas, and instructions in the *Mastering Motivation* chapter above.

- ***Finally, remember to use the BioSlim Formulas!*** They have been specifically formulated to help you in your battle against cravings. Do <u>not</u> rely on them exclusively, but rather use them as part of the entire BioSlim program. Their purpose is to help you fulfill the concepts and goals outlined here.

Remember: ultimately, it is the *whole program* that will work for you!

NINETEEN

MAINTAINING YOUR ACHIEVEMENTS
ଓଃଠ

When you've reached your health and weight goals, remember: **DON'T STOP FOLLOWING THE BIOSLIM SYSTEM!!** If there is one most important difference between this program and most others it is that BioSlim was *designed from the start to be permanent.* This is a lifelong way to stay healthy and at your proper weight. For it to work, you must continue to follow its main principles.

This does not mean that you must, for example, take the Formulas forever; they may be adjusted, or even stopped, as described earlier in the *BioSlim Formulas* chapter.

Nor does it mean that you must suffer in any way. In fact, the BioSlim program *depends* on your happiness.

You may also choose to "cheat" more often than you did during your losing phase. *But the basic program of eating (the Food Plan) and the Activity Plan should become a permanent part of your life.* This is the key to your long term success.

HOW IT'S DONE

- **KEEP UP YOUR FOOD PLAN, USE THE BIOSLIM COOKBOOK.** As you do, preparing food healthfully will become second nature to you. Soon you will be wondering how in the world you could ever cook and eat any other way, because you'll be feeling and looking so much better!

    The rewards that come from eating the old, unhealthful way are very transient indeed, lasting about as long as it takes to finish your meal. But the rewards of eating the BioSlim way—naturally, nutritiously, yet fully, with real, recognizable food—will last for the rest of your life. Every time you eat food that gives you pleasure and benefits you nutritionally at the same time, you'll be accomplishing something important that you can feel great about: your goal of having a healthy *and* attractive body, one that will be around a bit longer after each such accomplishment.

- Maintain your chosen **ACTIVITY PLAN**, as covered in the *Activity Plan* book.

- Take the **BIOSLIM FORMULAS** as per your needs. Each person decides what level of Formulas he or she needs to maintain good health and weight control once the initial goals are reached.

- **KEEP THIS BOOK ON YOUR BOOKSHELF PERMANENTLY** for reference whenever you have a question regarding health and fitness. You may well need it one day. Whether that day comes soon, or years from now—you will be glad you kept this book at the ready.

WE WANT YOU TO SUCCEED. PERMANENTLY.

That's what BioSlim is all about. And we'll do whatever we can to make sure you reach your goals — and keep them!

TWENTY

SOLVING PROBLEMS

I f you're like most people who experience the BioSlim system, you will meet with complete, ecstatic success.

Sometimes, however, you may come to believe that things should be going differently, or you may notice one of the special situations listed below. These occur because every human on this planet is different from every other. You are likely to react differently from anyone else to changes in your food intake, nutrition and activity level. Since every human is biologically unique, everyone starts with a personally defined metabolism and metabolic rate. Some may also have more digestive problems than others. Some may have a weak thyroid gland. Still others may be burdened with excess negative psychological baggage.

The following includes easy-to-implement, medically sound recommendations you can use to help overcome any challenges that appear:

I. WEIGHT LOSS IS TOO SLOW

VERY IMPORTANT POINT: *Everyone loses weight at his or her own individual pace!* You must remember this. Do not be overly concerned if you're losing weight at only a rate of, say, 1 pound per week, or even ½ pound per week. Experience has shown us that when weight loss is approached correctly, people can lose as much as 8-10 pounds per week or as little as ½ pound per week. These rates vary from week to week, month to month.

The important thing is to be going in the right direction. Your actual rate of weight loss depends on many distinctly personal, individualized factors, as listed below. Remember too that many people start slowly, picking up momentum as time goes on. Some people can take up to two months to "get up to speed". Finally, remember that if you are exercising, you may be losing lots of fat but not much weight, because you may be, for a while, replacing fat with toned muscle, which is heavier than fat.

Before reviewing the factors affecting your rate of weight loss, note this reminder: **IF YOU ARE NOT GETTING THE EFFECT YOU WANT, FIRST ADJUST YOUR DOSAGES OF THE FORMULAS,** using the instructions in the *BioSlim Formulas* chapter above. Of course, if you have not been using the Formulas correctly, do so. In any event, combine these actions with the information below to achieve optimal results.

(Also, consider adding an EFA (Essential Fatty Acid) supplement to your regimen. See the *BioSlim Formulas* chapter above for more information on this and other helpful concepts.)

Here are the various factors, concepts and tips that can affect your rate of weight loss:

- **YOUR STARTING POINT.** Often—but certainly not always—the more weight you need to lose, the *faster* you'll lose it in the beginning. If you need to lose 5 or 10 pounds, it's going to take a bit longer than the first 10 pounds in someone who needs to lose 100.

- **YOUR INDIVIDUAL BIOCHEMICAL, METABOLIC AND HORMONAL CONDITION.** You must make sure you don't have a medical, metabolic or hormonal problem. See the *Medical Considerations* section above. And remember to adjust your SlimTone Formula and Vita/Min Plus doses as detailed in *The BioSlim Formulas* chapter above.

- **HOW WELL YOU ADHERE TO THE FOOD PLAN.** This is a key factor, as some people "cheat" far too often during their weight-losing period, which inevitably slows down, and may well stop or *reverse* the process.

If cravings are the problem, see the *What To Do About Those Cravings* chapter above.

If eating in restaurants is the issue, see the *Restaurant Eating* section of the *BioSlim Food Plan* chapter above. The key here is **choosing from the menu only those foods that have no added fats or oils,** or at worst, just a little, and not overeating sugar and concentrated carbohydrate food. Dinner rolls smothered in butter are the *worst!* Choose restaurants that will comply with your desire to avoid health-destroying ingredients.

Finally, the *BioSlim CookBook* contains detailed alternatives to such things as oily salad dressings, ice cream, oil, etc., as well as a wide assortment of healthful, *delicious* food.

- **HOW ACTIVE YOU ARE.** The more the better. See the *Activity Plan* book and chapter above for more details.

- **YOUR FOOD TIMING.** If you're too busy, or if you forget to eat properly throughout the day only to come home in the evening to eat one huge meal for the day—you will not do as well as you would by *spreading out the food you eat* throughout the day. **BEST SUGGESTION:** Eat your largest meal at lunch, and your *lightest* meal for dinner. Also, have dinner as early as possible. Breakfast should be at least moderate, up to as much as you want to eat in the morning.

- **EAT SLOWLY.** Rapid eating *confuses* your internal sense of surfeit, making you much more likely to eat more than you really need. Try putting your utensils down after each bite, and not picking them up again until all the food is fully chewed and swallowed.

- <u>**EAT ONLY WHEN HUNGRY,**</u> not just because it's "lunch time" or "dinner time". Learn to recognize your body's signals of true versus false hunger. (See above, *Mastering Motivation*)

- **STOP EATING WHEN YOU'RE NO LONGER HUNGRY.** For most of us, this is very hard to do because we are trained in childhood to *finish what's in front of us*. Breaking that lifelong habit can be very difficult—but very rewarding, as this is precisely what *naturally* thin people do, and it is how nature intended for us to eat. (See *Mastering Motivation*)

- If you cannot find a way to stop eating when no longer hungry, **THINK ABOUT WHETHER YOU'RE TRULY HUNGRY OR NOT.** If you're not sure, *you're not!* Hunger is obvious, a *physical* feeling. It is not mistakable, once you learn to recognize it. (Also note: you may simply be *thirsty!*)

- **TRY WRITING DOWN**, on a small pad of paper you carry with you, everything that is about to enter your mouth just beforeit enters it, but after you've made the decision to eat it. This action alone causes weight loss! (See the *Mastering Motivation* and *Cravings* chapters above for more ways to help.)

IF YOU'VE DONE EVERYTHING ELSE and you're still not losing weight fast enough, remember that it is possible you have reached your optimal weight. Most people should not try to be rail-thin. This media image of "perfection" is both impossible and dangerous for most people to try to achieve. Each of us has a natural, optimal weight level below which we become *less* healthy. Do not cross that line.

Ia. WHEN TO USE *SUPER BIOSLIM*

This special plan, described in the *Appendix* of this book, should be used if the standard BioSlim Plan as described so far is not enough to get you started on the path of true weight control. Super BioSlim is very powerful, and much more intensive than the regular plan. It is not meant to be continued permanently, not because it is unhealthful—it is *extremely* healthful. But it is also simply too difficult for most people to maintain. The primary purpose of *Super BioSlim* is to help people who are having a difficult time getting started. If you choose to use this plan, eventually you will have to decide on a *permanent* system for yourself, which can be the standard BioSlim program, or some combination of *Super BioSlim* and standard BioSlim. The best program is the one you know you can stick with.

II. WEIGHT LOSS IS TOO RAPID

Most people would not consider this a problem. However, if your rapid weight loss is being achieved through near-starvation, or through some strange, unnaturally restrictive "diet", or through the use of diet powder or diet shakes—STOP! This is definitely *not* what BioSlim is about, and *not* the way to lose weight healthfully and permanently. If you're doing this, be aware that your weight will probably come back.

On the other hand, if you're losing weight rapidly because you're following the Food Plan (or the *Super BioSlim* Plan) closely, getting plenty of activity, and taking your Formulas as directed—*keep it up!* The number of pounds you lose per week is *not* the deciding factor in determining whether you're doing it right or not. It's how good you're being to your body that counts!

As usual, check with your doctor if anything unusual occurs.

III. ENERGY LEVEL IS NOT HIGH ENOUGH

BioSlim is designed to help improve your energy level. If this is not happening for you, do the following:

- **MAKE SURE YOU DO NOT HAVE A MEDICAL PROBLEM.** Check with your doctor if your symptoms are unusual.
- **WAIT.** It can take up to 1-2 months in some cases for the full benefits of the system to be fully realized.
- **INCREASE THE DOSAGE OF SLIMTONE FORMULA.** Follow the guidelines listed in the *BioSlim Formulas* chapter above.
- **MAKE SURE** you're on full dose **VITA/MIN PLUS**.
- **ARE YOU ACTIVE ENOUGH?**
- **ARE YOU "CHEATING" ON THE BIOSLIM FOOD PLAN?** You would be amazed how sometimes even a little

cheating (especially with foods high in fat, oil or sugar) can affect your overall sense of well-being and energy level.

- **TRY CUTTING OUT ALL MILK PRODUCTS.** For many reasons, including widespread milk sensitivities, milk causes many problems for many people. Try cutting it out completely. (A good substitute is vanilla-, chocolate- or carob-flavored soy-milk, available at health stores.)
- **IF YOU'VE DONE EVERYTHING RIGHT:** I.e., if you've waited the recommended length of time and followed all aspects of the BioSlim program, and still feel the need for improved energy—go back and review the *Medical Considerations* chapter above; you may find something you missed earlier. Then check with your doctor for any metabolic, biochemical, hormonal, hematological, or other organic problem you may be experiencing that may be causing your lack of energy.

IV. ENERGY LEVEL IS TOO HIGH

If you're having trouble sleeping, or if you are simply becoming too "energetic":

- **DON'T TAKE YOUR BIOSLIM FORMULAS TOO CLOSE TO BEDTIME.** The Vita/Min Plus tabs, for example can be taken at breakfast and at lunch, while the SlimTone Formula can be similarly taken twice *or* three times per day, with the last dose coming well before dinnertime.
- **WAIT.** This effect usually dissipates within two weeks.
- **IF YOU'VE WAITED LONG ENOUGH,** try *reducing* your SlimTone Formula dosage as described in the appropriate sections above.
- **NEXT, TRY REDUCING** Vita/Min Plus as described earlier.
- **IF NONE OF THIS WORKS,** check with your doctor for any medical problem that may be causing this effect.
- **AND IF NONE OF THE ABOVE PROVIDES A SOLUTION,** and your doctor doesn't think there's a problem, you should

probably stop worrying about it. This may be your *normal* state—something you are simply not used to yet. Energy!

V. YOUR DIGESTIVE TRACT

- CONSTIPATION OR DIARRHEA

This can result from any change of eating habits. Occasionally, the BioSlim Formulas may cause some bowel loosening, though this effect is usually very mild. Remember: proper bowel function is important to health and weight maintenance, and that means moving your bowels at least once per day, though two, three, or even four times per day is perfectly healthful, as long as the movements are not diarrheal (watery).

If you're experiencing constipation, make sure to drink *plenty* of water (that's water, not juice) during the day. Of course, you should be doing this anyway on the BioSlim System (see the *Food Plan* chapter above); but it is even more essential if your bowels are a bit slow. Remember: The most common cause of constipation is insufficient water intake.

Also, be sure to eat lots of **FIBER**. Fiber not only *regulates* the bowels (it helps control *both* diarrhea and constipation!), it may also help prevent certain forms of cancer and heart disease. It's definitely something you want to get plenty of! Fiber is found in virtually all non-animal foods: vegetables, fruit, whole grains, etc. It is virtually **absent** in all animal products such as milk and milk products, meat, fish, chicken, eggs, etc., and in refined, processed foods like white bread, white sugar, white rice. If you take fiber supplements, you must drink lots of water too!

Finally, if constipation persists beyond 1-2 weeks, consider trying some magnesium citrate or milk of magnesia once or twice to get things moving; use as directed on the bottle or jar.

Consult your physician if anything unusual occurs.

- INTESTINAL GAS

This too occurs with greater frequency when diet is changed in any way. Increasing fiber intake (see above paragraph) is a particularly common reason for this symptom. The solution is to WAIT. It will probably pass within two weeks or so. If not, try adjusting your meals so that they are *simpler,* by not mixing sweets with other foods, avoiding desserts altogether, minimizing juices and soft drinks taken with meals and avoiding the combination of fruit with meats and starchy foods. The idea is to eat simple meals that consist of related, like-digestible foods. A *lactobacillus* supplement (see *Colitis* in the *Medical Considerations* chapter above) should also be very helpful.

VI. WHEN TO SEE YOUR DOCTOR

In general, see your doctor if any physical symptom or sign occurs that is unusual or makes you uncomfortable or worried in any way! Also, see above, and see the chapter on *Medical Considerations* for many references to specific issues.

TWENTY-ONE

WOMEN: SPECIAL FACTS AND CONSIDERATIONS

☙❧

♀

Women have certain unique requirements, varying with age. Here are a few of the issues women face, and how the BioSlim system impacts them.

THE THYROID: NOTHING WORKS IF IT DOES NOT

Women are far more likely to have a disorder involving this vital hormone-producing gland than men. See *Thyroid Gland Disease* in the *Medical Considerations* chapter above for more information on symptoms, testing and treatment.

Most important to remember: You must know for sure that your thyroid gland is working properly. If you suspect you may have this kind of problem, get tested, and if necessary, treated. *If your thyroid is not working properly, unless you receive proper treatment not even the BioSlim program will help you lose weight and become healthier.* The thyroid gland produces hormones that function as master regulators for the whole body; it is vitally important that these hormones function properly.

SPECIAL NUTRITIONAL REQUIREMENTS

Protein requirements are typically *lower* for women compared to men, as are calorie requirements. This latter point means that on average, women must eat *less* food in order to maintain their weight as compared to men.

After adjustment for weight, women often need *more* vitamin B6, folic acid, calcium, magnesium, and iron than do men. Women also often require more EFAs (Essential Fatty Acids).

The BioSlim program includes a balance of nutrients appropriate for most women. Some individuals may wish to add:

- Extra calcium and magnesium, particularly after menopause. (Reasonable *additional* daily amounts: 750 and 500 mg, respectively.)
- Extra iron, but only if iron-deficiency is proven with a fasting blood test. (Normal dose for women: 18 mg/day, or as directed by doctor.) See below under *Iron/Anemia*.
- Extra folic acid if it is possible that pregnancy may occur, or if cervical dysplasia (abnormal cells in the uterine cervix) is discovered. (For potential pregnancy: extra 400 to 600 mcg per day, for a daily total of 800 to 1000 mcg; for cervical dysplasia: extra 2000 to 3000 mcg per day.)
- Essential Fatty Acids, particularly if suffering from dry skin or hair, weak or brittle nails, menstrual difficulties, mood swings, arthritis, et al, as discussed in the *Nutrition: The Key to Health* chapter above.

THE BODY

Women naturally have more body fat, measured as a percentage of total body mass, than do men. Often this fat is distributed in places considered aesthetically undesirable. But regardless of what we think of it, this is nature's reality. For most women, it is unnatural and nearly *impossible* to attain the ultra-thin appearance of professional models. It is best not to try. Maximize the body you were born with but do not try to accomplish that which is unhealthy and unnatural.

IRON / ANEMIA

Women are far more likely to be anemic than men, mostly because of menstruation.

MOST IMPORTANT TO REMEMBER: Get checked, particularly if you have unexpected fatigue, pallor, heavy bleeding, and any of the other symptoms and signs described under *Anemia* in the *Medical Considerations* chapter above.

Remember too that anemia does *not* equal iron deficiency. Anemia means there is a deficiency of hemoglobin and/or red blood cells. Iron deficiency means what it says: a shortage in the body of the mineral iron. Iron deficiency is the most common *cause* of anemia, since iron is required for the formation of hemoglobin, the molecules inside red blood cells. But it is not the only cause, and it is *not* synonymous with the term anemia.

If you are anemic, it is vital to take a good multi-nutrient formula, like BioSlim Vita/Min Plus. Consideration should also be given to extra iron supplementation, at least until blood iron and red cell levels are normalized (see *Special Nutritional Requirements* above for dosages).

PREGNANCY

While the **Vita/Min Plus** multi-vitamin-mineral tabs *may* be used during pregnancy, they are not recommended. Your doctor-recommended, or health-store-bought PRENATAL nutritional supplements are best.

And though **SlimTone Formula** is perfectly safe in general, pregnancy is definitely NOT the time to try to lose weight. Therefore, we recommend that you:

- **Follow your doctor's advice**
- **Follow the recommended BioSlim Food Plan.** It's the *healthiest* way to eat, and both you and your baby will benefit from it
- **Stop the BioSlim Formulas and switch to** PRENATAL nutritional supplementation

- **Check with your doctor** regarding your activity level

You may begin following the full BioSlim program anytime after you deliver.

MENSTRUAL CHANGES

It is very common for women to experience changes in their patterns of menstruation as a result of such things as: stress, change in diet, excessive exercise, and many other factors that may come up in a woman's life. Of course, if *anything* unusual or worrisome is going on, check with your doctor. But typically, this change will settle out within one or two cycles.

Many women report a *normalization* of menstrual cycles and symptoms on the BioSlim program. This is one of those *side benefits* we spoke of earlier. Enjoy it!

MENOPAUSE

Menopause is a natural change of life that every woman must experience. It is *not* a disease.

Whether or not to use hormone replacement therapy (estrogen, and possibly progesterone pills) is a decision you must make with your personal physician. But in the absence of disturbing menopausal symptoms, it is important to recognize that menopause is a perfectly normal part of life. In my view, things unbroken should not be fixed, particularly when the repair-people understand so little of the true mechanisms by which the whole organism works.

MOST IMPORTANT TO REMEMBER: (a) Take extra calcium and magnesium supplementation, as described above; (b) stay active! Nothing is more effective at keeping a woman young, healthy, and non-osteoporotic (i.e., with strong bones) than plenty of physical activity. Do as much as prudence and medical considerations permit.

YEAST SYNDROMES

Yeast infections are extremely common in women. See *Vaginitis* in the *Medical Considerations* chapter above for more information on symptoms, testing and the treatment of the most common manifestation of yeast infection.

There has been considerable controversy over the possible existence of something called the *yeast* or *candida syndrome*. This has been proposed by some as a cause of a very large, diverse number of disease and disorders, mostly of the chronic variety. Examples include: chronic fatigue, menstrual problems, arthritis, headaches, assorted allergic symptoms, weakened immune system, and many others. The syndrome is described as being caused by an overgrowth of yeast, mostly in the intestinal and vaginal areas, which is hypothesized as causing disease through allergies and "toxins".

Unfortunately, there is very little real evidence to support the hypothesis that yeast actually *causes* any of the disorders with which it has been associated. The ground on which this theory's proponents stand is far, far shakier than, for example, the ground on which the HIV-causes-AIDS hypothesis stands. In both cases, it has never been proven that the organism in question actually *causes* the disease(s) with which it is associated. (Just because many people with AIDS carry the HIV virus does *not* prove that HIV causes AIDS, though it is certainly likely.) To a far greater degree, just because *some* people with chronic fatigue, menstrual difficulties, headaches, and many other disorders have yeast in their bodies—does not in any way prove that yeast *causes* anything. Keep in mind that a small amount of yeast is normal in the human gut and vagina.

This syndrome is often diagnosed with *no evidence at all* beyond simple conjecture and the highly unscientific "tests" (actually questionnaires) published in popular books.

It is very likely that the presence of an overgrowth of yeast is a *marker*, or sign, of the presence of weakened defenses. That is, it is a symptom or sign that appears *because of some other underlying problem or deficiency,* rather than being itself a primary cause of disease. Once present though, chronic yeast overgrowth can become a significant exacerbating factor.

The approach to yeast infections is described above under *Vaginitis* in the *Medical Considerations* chapter. The most important preventive measures are: (a) avoid tight, synthetic clothing; (b) avoid excessive sweets and all junk food; (c) practice excellent hygiene, and insist that your partner do so as well; (d) take supplemental *lactobacillus* (described earlier); (e) consider taking oral medication against yeast, such as *Nystatin* and others, in addition to topical treatments, and (f) if you get treated, be sure your partner gets treated simultaneously, so that you do not end up transmitting the infection back and forth.

TWENTY-TWO

THE FUTURE
ଔଊ

As you get closer to your goals and ultimately achieve them, always remember that this is not a short-term experience. Your *real* goal is a *permanent* change in your life.

As you succeed, your friends and family will want to know how you did it.

How *you* did it.

Tell them how *you* did it. How you did not need any gimmicks, or anyone standing over you telling you what to do. How you simply let your body follow a natural, healthful path to better health and a leaner profile.

You are in charge, you are the one who can and will reach all your goals. As you look to the future, remind yourself of all you have done and all that you will do. And let BioSlim help you— take from the program everything you possibly can.

If you have thoughts, comments or questions concerning the program, please write to us at BioSlim. We are always looking for ways to enhance and improve the program, and there is nothing more important to that process than your feelings, opinions and reactions.

Speaking for myself and for all of us at BioSlim, we wish you the very best of health.

J. Leichtberg, M.D.
and the BioSlim staff

SECTION THREE

APPENDIX

FOODS AT A GLANCE
ॐ

Please see Chapter 12 and the BioSlim CookBook for much more information regarding food, and many ideas and tips on what to eat and when. Here's a quick overview of the BioSlim food plan, along with suggestions for specific foods to eat and menus to follow at various times of the day. (You may, of course, eat any of these foods with any meal.)

Remember, *you are in charge!* You choose which way you want to eat, using our ideas, menus and recipes as guidelines. The BioSlim CookBook is a terrific resource for food ideas that will satisfy you and keep you going on the BioSlim System.

(Note: The CookBook contains a few recipes that are marked for use during the maintenance phase of weight control. These should be avoided during the losing phase, or altered to reduce fat and/or concentrated carbohydrate levels.)

GENERAL GUIDELINES REVIEW:

1. Don't add oil, butter, margarine, mayonnaise or any <u>added fat</u> to your food!

2. Do your best to minimize **flour products**, such as bread, all pasta and cakes. When you do eat flour products, <u>in moderation,</u> make sure it is made with whole grain, such 100% whole wheat.

3. Be wary of rice, potatoes, corn and carrot—these are all high-carbohydrate (starchy) foods that should be balanced with protein foods. White rice should be avoided altogether; it is equivalent to white flour (which is used to make white bread and pasta)—nutritionally empty, fat-building high-carbohydrate food.

4. Best avoid those high-sugar soft drinks. (Remember, sugar is a carbohydrate, and also needs to be protein-balanced.) Diet drinks are OK, but like all else, use moderation. Remember that fruit juices are also very high in sugar (carbohydrate), and should be moderated—best diluted at least 50:50 with water.

5. Eat equal portions of high-carbohydrate food (all flour products, all sweet food, potatoes, carrots—see below for complete list) and high-protein foods (meat, fish, chicken, turkey, eggs, non-fat milk, non-or-low-fat cheese, soy products, spirulina—see below for list). You need not bother weighing anything. The best and easiest approach is to make "eyeball" judgments. On average, this will work just as well as weighing. For example, if you are having oatmeal, or a small piece of (whole grain) bread, add a few slices of chicken or turkey, or some eggs or egg whites.

6. Milk and milk products are OK if they are non-fat or low-fat (assuming you are not allergic or otherwise intolerant, of course).

7. Drink at least six to eight 12-ounce glasses of water per day.

8. It is best to avoid eating very large meals—better to spread food out through your day. Also, try to eat small dinners and avoid eating within 2 hours of bedtime.

9. Use the BioSlim Formulas as directed. Be as active as you can be. And follow the BioSlim program as closely as possible.

SAMPLES: QUICK SNACKS

1. Fat-free turkey or chicken deli slices. Tomato & cucumber with balsamic vinegar or lemon juice + salt, with some low-fat crackers.

2. Turkey slices rolled up in lettuce leaf with salsa inside.

3. Tuna packed in water (NOT OIL), plus tomato, pickles, lettuce.

4. 1-2 eggs, hard boiled or any other way, plus any vegetable, such as fresh, frozen or canned asparagus, artichoke hearts (frozen or canned, in water not oil), peas and beans, etc.

5. Low or non-fat cottage cheese plus piece of fruit (see below).

6. Turkey slices wrapped around a low-fat cracker with celery or other vegetable.

7. Canned artichoke hearts (packed in water, not oil) plus (fat-free) salsa. A delicious combination, filling yet fat-friendly.

8. Open a can of asparagus, available in any supermarket. It's delicious, fast and filling. Try the same with other green vegetables, frozen or canned: spinach, broccoli, green beans, etc. Combine with any protein food listed below, most easily those delicious thin-sliced fat-free turkey or chicken slices available in your supermarket's deli section.

SAMPLES: GOOD BREAKFAST CHOICES

1. Eggs (especially egg whites), oatmeal or whole-grain toast, non-fat milk or low-fat soymilk, vegetable (tomato, cucumber, celery)

2. Oatmeal with skim milk plus non-fat turkey/chicken deli slices.

3. Vegetables (salad, tomato, cucumber, celery, asparagus, artichoke, broccoli, etc.) plus chicken or turkey breast or deli slices.

4. Low-fat or non-fat yogurt plus bran cereal or oatmeal.

5. Any combination of the QUICK SNACKS above.

6. Blended spirulina (see page 121 for more information). Rinse it down with water, herbal tea, or diluted fruit juice.

7. *Blended Salad* from the CookBook, plus smoked fat-free turkey deli slices.

8. Large salad with fat-free dressing (see *BioSlim CookBook* for recipes). Add chopped or sliced hard-boiled eggs for protein.

SAMPLES: LUNCH and DINNER

1. Chicken breast prepared without added fat, plus any green vegetable (broccoli, asparagus, spinach, beans, etc.) Fruit optional.

2. Fish prepared without added fat, plus green vegetable of your choice (broccoli, asparagus, spinach, beans, etc.)

3. Egg omelet (no high-fat cheese or oil), prepared with vegetables.

4. Turkey burger plus salad (no oil) and green vegetable of your choice. Fruit optional.

5. Soy or vegi-burger, plus hard boiled egg (white-only or whole) and salad.

6. Eggplant parmigiana made with low-fat or fat-free cheese. Add some turkey or chicken deli slices for extra protein, plus salad and green vegetable of your choice.

7. Chicken or turkey breast (prepared without added oil or fat) plus *Lively Lentil Taco* from the CookBook.

8. *Don't-Be-A-Turkey Loaf* or *Turkey Burger* (from the Cook-Book), plus salad and/or green vegetables, topped with some fruit.

9. Any CookBook soup, plus egg, turkey or chicken for protein.

10. *Mom's Eggplant Ecstasy* from the CookBook, plus extra egg or turkey slices, and tomato and cucumber on the side.

11. *Tasty Tomato Soup* plus *Great Garlic Turkey Breast* plus *Green Bean Tomato Sidekick*, all from the CookBook.

12. *Vegetable Turkey Or Chicken Breasts* plus *Oh How Sweet Pea Soup* (from the CookBook) and any green vegetable.

13. *Turkey Enchilada Casserole, Leading Lentil Soup* plus *Vibrant Vegetable Circus* (see CookBook) and a tossed salad.

14. Fat free hot-dogs (soy or regular), plus *Okra Gumbo Soup* (see CookBook).

15. *Gala Gaspacho Soup* plus *Mexican Chicken Salad* (see CookBook) plus vegetable salad (see CookBook for fat-free dressings).

16. Any combination of the QUICK SNACKS above.

VEGETABLES:
Raw, frozen, steamed, or canned. Avoid or minimize potato, carrot and beet as these are very high-carbohydrate foods (high in starch),

and should always be eaten in moderation and balanced with protein. Examples of "good" vegetables (or beans and lentils) which may be eaten in virtually *any* reasonable quantity:
• Brussels sprouts, Broccoli, Cauliflower
• All green leafy vegetables, e.g. spinach/kale, any lettuce, etc.
• Radish, Tomato, Cucumber, Celery, Salsa
• Sprouts
• Peas, Zucchini, Squash
• Lentils, Beans (no oil or lard added, of course), in moderation
• Or any combination of the above from the frozen-food section of your food store.

FRUITS:
Avoid or minimize banana, grape, raisin, watermelon—these are very high-carbohydrate foods (high in sugar) and should always be eaten in moderation and balanced with protein. In general, **do not overdo fruits**, especially those that are loaded with sugar (i.e., very sweet). The best fruits are the least sweet and juiciest, e.g., grapefruit, or even pineapple. Berries and cherries are also usually fine.

HIGH-PROTEIN FOODS:
All items should be prepared without added oil or fat.
• Chicken or turkey FAT-FREE deli slices (pure protein)
• Chicken or turkey breast, skinless
• Eggs, especially egg whites, which are pure protein and can be eaten in any reasonable quantity
• Fish, Seafood
• Milk, non-fat or very-low-fat Cheese, Yogurt
• Soy products, such as soymilk, soy-burgers, non-or-low-fat soy hot-dogs, non-or-low-fat soy deli slices, etc.
• Spirulina
• Occasional piece of very low-fat beef

HIGH-CARBOHYDRATE FOODS:
These are to be either avoided or minimized. When consumed, they should be balanced (by eyeballing, or visually approximating

the relative weights of the amounts to be consumed) with high protein food. The list below is in descending order, i.e., the first ones on this list are the most important to avoid.
- **All flour products**, including bread, pasta, cake, cookies, pizza, etc. When you do consume flour products, look for whole grain flour, and balance them with high-protein food.
- **Sugar**, in all its forms. This includes sweet foods such as banana, grapes, raisins, soft drinks, undiluted fruit juice, in addition to the obvious: all manner of candy, cookies and cakes.
- Potato and rice, especially white rice
- Corn, Carrot, Beet

FAST FOOD OUTLETS:
See also above under QUICK SNACKS.
- Lean Cuisine is fine, but avoid the pastas and other high-flour products.
- McDonald's — Salads (without the cheese), eggs
- Taco Bell — Light chicken tacos, eggs, other low-fat, low carbohydrate food
- Any diner or luncheonette — eggs, chicken or turkey breast, fish, seafood, salads, any of the vegetables listed above.

TIPS:
- Oil or butter substitute: Chicken broth, water or tomato sauce
- Substitute for cream: Evaporated non-fat milk. Milk or soymilk. Cashews, ground with water.
- Seasonings: Vinegar, all kinds: best are balsamic and rice wine. Lemon juice. Mustard. Soy sauce. Bragg's (low sodium soy sauce substitute).
- Salt: may be eaten in any reasonable quantity, assuming you are not told differently by your physician. Seasoning salt is particularly good on salads with balsamic vinegar or lemon juice. Best seasoning salt: Herbamare.

THE SUPER BIOSLIM PLAN

This is a special new addition to BioSlim. It incorporates a more intensive food plan than standard BioSlim, and is designed for use by those individuals who do not readily or easily find success under the standard program.

Super BioSlim is not designed to be adopted as a permanent plan. It is, rather, a limited-term way to "get the ball rolling", to help those who need more help get started on the path to true weight control. This is not because *Super BioSlim* is in any way unhealthful—it is <u>*extremely*</u> healthful. But it is also simply too difficult for most people to maintain over long periods of time.

If you choose to use this plan, eventually you should decide on a *permanent* system for yourself. This can be the standard BioSlim program, or some <u>combination</u> of *Super BioSlim* and standard BioSlim. The best program will be the one you know you can stick with. The key word here is: *permanent*.

Super BioSlim can also be used to achieve very rapid weight loss by anyone, without even trying the standard BioSlim plan. It is recognized that some people will do this. If you are one, remember again that *Super BioSlim* is not meant as a permanent solution to the weight control dilemma. It is a powerful "quick fix" beginning. We do not expect you to necessarily stay on it forever. A permanent program must still be adopted if you are to avoid the unfortunately all-too-familiar "yo-yo" phenomenon.

How *Super BioSlim* Works

The use of the BioSlim Formulas remains unchanged. Follow the instructions previously outlined.

The Activity Plan also remains unchanged, though for best results it is recommended that you do your activities as often and as intensively (but safely!) as you can. Push it, for best results.

The key difference between the standard BioSlim Plan and *Super BioSlim* is in what you eat. Control over your food plan must be tighter under this plan than under the regular plan.

SPECIFICALLY ELIMINATED ARE:

- **ALL** fats and oils (not just the *added* kind as in regular BioSlim). In addition to what should be avoided in the standard BioSlim Food Plan, also avoid or minimize natural high-fat foods such as: peanut butter, marbled meat, egg yolk, fatty fish or seafood, avocado, sesame seeds, tahini, etc. In short, anything that contains excessive fat or oil.
- ALL sweets, all sugars. And any food that contains anything more than a little sugar. Avoid fruit juices. And minimize anything more than occasional sweet fruit.
- ALL concentrated high-carbohydrate foods, both starchy and sweet. This is a key point, vital to the success of the plan. It means avoiding (or severely minimizing): bread, pasta, *all* flour products, potatoes, rice, corn, bananas, carrots, beets raisins, grapes. Focus on high protein food. Under *Super BioSlim*, you need not necessarily balance all protein with equivalent amounts of carbohydrates. You may tip the balance in favor of protein. Do *not*, however, eat *more* carbohydrates than protein!

WHAT TO EAT:

Eat high protein, low-fat items that do not contain concentrated starch or sweets. Examples:

- All vegetables, other than those listed above. All green vegetables may be eaten at will. Asparagus, fresh, frozen or

- canned, broccoli, cauliflower, artichoke (in water) and Brussels sprouts are examples of some of the best choices.
- Egg whites—may be eaten at will. Try, for example, using several hard-boiled egg whites instead of pasta with some fat-free tomato sauce. It's delicious!
- Fat-free deli slices made from meat or from soy. The soy varieties are particularly interesting, since they can be obtained truly fat-free, are often just as delicious as the real thing, and they contain fiber, something no animal product can claim.
- Spirulina. This is highly recommended for breakfast. You may blend it in the morning with your vitamins and get it all over with in a matter of minutes. (Some juice is OK to use for killing that "wonderful" spirulina flavor.) If you must chew on something, eat fat-free deli slices and/or any green vegetable as a chaser.
- Occasional low-fat fish or fowl (white meat only) is OK, in moderation.
- DRINK PLENTY OF WATER! This is a VITAL element of the plan. Drink fresh, clean water all day long. Especially if you feel a craving coming on. Do NOT drink fruit juices, milk, soft drinks, etc.

Is it easy?

Super BioSlim is not meant to be easy. It's meant to be powerful—the most powerful plan you can be on.

So you may find it challenging to stick with it for long. That's why it is not considered truly permanent. But if you want results, especially if you've had trouble getting started on standard BioSlim, this is the ultimate game plan. It pulls no punches.

Remember: The closer you follow this plan, the faster your weight will come off. The more you cut corners, the more you compromise, the slower will be your results. Consider this simple one-to-one relationship between plan elements and weight loss results a certainty. If you really mean to get results this time, do it all! Be perfect!

Once you've begun losing weight, start thinking about what kind of *permanent* plan you can live with. Compare the elements of *Super BioSlim* with the standard BioSlim Food Plan and decide for yourself which parts of which plan you want to live with permanently. Then switch to that permanent plan when you're ready, which will probably be either (a) when you have reached your weight goal or (b) when you feel you can no longer find the motivation to continue the powerful but challenging *Super BioSlim* plan.

And remember: your transition should be smooth and easy, so that your weight losing process continues unabated.

INDEX

Abbott Laboratories, 21
abdominal pain, 56, 59, 96
Abraham Lincoln, 92
absorption, 127, 128
acetyl-CoA, 25
achievements, maintaining, 189
acidophilus, 71, 98
Activity Plan, 63, **152**, 190
   benefits of, 153
   diet and, 154
   rules of, 155
acupuncture, 65, 79, 93
Acutrim, 26
added fats, 103, 186, 207
adipocytes. *See* fat cells
adrenal, 85
   insufficiency, 36, 56
   gland dysfunction, 56
aging, 14, 17, 57
   slowing down, 57, 58
AIDS, 75, 203
air pollution, asthma and, 88
alcohol, 71, 89, 184
   occasional use, 117
   pregnancy and, 90
   ulcer disease and, 97
alfalfa sprouts, 105
alkylglycerols, 64
allergies, 58, 203
   food, 58, 181, 183
   food, testing for, 58
almonds, 86
aloe vera, 97

alternative therapies, 64
amaranth, 115
Americans, % overweight, 4
amino acids, 130
   essential, 130
anemia, **59**, 61, 75, 79, 96, 201
   iron deficiency &, 60, 201
   thyroid disorders and, 94
   women and, **201**
angelica sin., & headaches, 80
anger, 16
angina, 81
anthropometry, 8
antibiotics, **35-38**, 71, 86
   in children, 36
   microbial resistance to, 37
   overuse of, 37
antihistamines, 13
antioxidants, **57-58**, 64, 140
   and aging, 57
anxiety, 94
appetite, 33
   loss of, 59
appetite control center, 16
apple cider vinegar, 62, 113
Armour Thyroid, 95
arrhythmias, 23, 83
arthritis, **60**, 203
asparagus, 209, 214
aspartic acid, 78
aspirin, 143
astemizole, 13
asthma, **62**, 86, 87

217

atherosclerosis, 18, **82-83**
Atkins diet, 20, **24**
  side effects, 25
atrophic vaginitis, 98
Augmentin, 36
auto-immune disorders, 61
  and fatigue, 76
avocado, 15

B complex, 137
B vitamins, 59, 78, 93, **137**, 147
back pain, **62**, 96
bacteria, 37
  beneficial/friendly, 38, 71, 78, 97-98
banana, 107, 211-12
barley, 71
bars, diet, 10, 20, 22, 24, 31, 101
basal body temperature test for thyroid, 94
basal metabolism, 13
  effect of activity on, 13
basic food groups, 3
beans, 112, 208-9, 211
beef, 211
beer, 185
beet, 14, 212
beet greens, 105
beta carotene, 121, 136
biofeedback, 79
  high blood pressure &, 85
  stress and, 92
bioflavonoids, 59, 62, 65, 84, 97, **140**
BioSlim
  Activity Plan, 63
  aging and, 57
  anti-cancer aspects of, 64
  changing your life with, 49
  cholesterol lowering &, 68-69
  chronic fatigue, in, 77
  combined with drug(s), 26
  defined, 29
  development of, 35
  Food Plan, 58, 69, 102, 103, 182, 207
  future and, 205
  heart health and, 82
  helping achieve goals, 47
  keeping it simple, 11
  medical considerations, 53
  medical group and, 35
  medications and, 56
  options before, 20
  preventing diabetes, 73
  Principles of, 103
  saving money with, 33
  side benefits from, 34
  staying happy, 51
  thyroid disorders and, 96
  ulcer disease and, 98
  what it is and is not, 50
  what it's about, 5
  your goals with, 32
BioSlim Formulas, 28, 32-33, 49, 57, 59-60, 62, 64, 66, 69, 73, 77-8, 80, 83-4, 86, 88, 90, 93, 97, 129, 139, 142, **145**, 146, 182-3, 188, 192, 196, 208
  and pregnancy, 91
biotin, 138
Biotique skin care, 92
birth control pills, 79
blood clots, 18
blood pressure, 56
  high, 14, 18
  low, 56

blood sugar, 6, 56, 181
   high, 56
blue-green algae, 121, 130
BMI. *See Body Mass Index*
body fat analysis, 8, 11
Body Mass Index, 9
bone density, 153
bone marrow, 59
bowel habits, 33
Bragg's, 212
bread, 6, 14, 114, 197, 207, 212
breakfast, 209
breakfast, importance of, 109
breast cancer
   estrogen and, 89
breast feeding, 38
   BioSlim Formulas and, 91
breathing disorders, 18
broccoli, 105, 209, 211, 215
bromelain, 64, 83, 151
bronchi, 87
bronchitis, 37, 86
Brussels sprouts, 211, 215
buckwheat, 115
butter, 116, 185, 207

cabbage, 105
   extract, & peptic ulcers, 97
caffeine, 79, 120, 143, 144, 182
   addiction to, 79
   headaches and, 79
calcium, 59, 71, 77, 80, 90, 93, **141**, 147, 150, 200
calcium ascorbate, 139
California Slim, 22
calories, **129**
cancer, 3, 14, 18, 46, **63**, 68, 75, 76, 89, 117
   vitamin D and, 139
candida, 77, 98, 203

candies, 41, 117
canola oil, 15
caprylic acid, 98
carbohydrate intolerance, 13-14
carbohydrates, 6, 13, 14, 15, 42, 106, **131**, 186, 208
   balanced with proteins, 42
   complex, 132
   effect on blood sugar, 14
   effect on insulin levels, 14
   intolerance, 13-14
   puffed, 107
cardiovascular disease, 31, 81
carotenemia, 136
carotenes, 136
carpal tunnel syndrome, 65
carrot, 14, 107, 207-8, 212
cashews, 86, 212
cataracts, 65
cauliflower, 105, 211, 215
CCK, *See* cholecystokinin
celery, 105, 211
cellular respiration, 59
cereals, 41, 118
CFIDS, 77
chamomile, 113
chard, swiss, 105
cheating, 110, **124**, 195
cheese, 117, 185, 208, 211
chemotherapy, 63
cherries, 211
chicken, 72, 106, 111, 197, 208-9, 211-12
childhood obesity, 39
childhood, eating habits in, 16
chips, 41, 117
chiropractor, 9, 63
chives, 105
chlorella, 121
chocolate, 86, **118**, 185

cholangitis, 78
cholecystitis, 78
cholecystokinin, 15
cholesterol, 3, 7, 111, 133
    ages relevant to, 67
    diet and, 67
    drugs that lower, 67
    futility of reducing, 68
    HDL and, 67
    heart disease and, 66
    high, 18, 66
    lab tests for, 67
    LDL and, 67
    low level, 67
    manufactured by body, 66
    over-emphasis on, 66
    thyroid, 67
choline, 138
chromium, 69, 83, **142**
chronic fatigue syndrome, 76, 77
CFIDS, 77
Cipro, 36
circulation, 153
cocoa, 86, 118
coenzyme Q10, 143
coenzymes, 135
coffee, 120, 185
cold, sensitivity to, 94
colitis, 69
    cigarette smoking and, 70
    milk products and, 70
comfrey, 97
complex carbohydrates, 132
constipation, 25, **72**, 94, 197
    activity and, 72
    headaches and, 80
    hemorrhoids and, 84
    water and, 72

CookBook, 41, 104, 120, 189, 207, 209-10
cookies, 117, 212
COPD. *See* Chronic Obstructive Pulmonary Disease
copper, 60, 90, **142**
CoQ10, 69, 78, 83, 143
corn, 6, 14, 37, 71, 107, 115, 207, 212
    chips, 117
coronary arteries, 81
corticosteroids, 13
cosmetic surgery, 27
cravings, 25, **180**
    due to depression, 182
    due to food allergies, 183
    due to hypoglycemia, 181
    due to nutrition, 183
    food/diet imbalance, 184
    meal size and, 187
    physical reasons for, 181
    prevent and stop, 185
    psychological vs. physical, 180
    sugar and, 186
    thyroid dysfunction, 182
    tooth brushing and, 187
    water and, 186
cream cheese, 41, 117
cucumber, 105, 208, 210-11
Cushing's syndrome, 56
cystine, 86

dandelion, 86
death, sudden, 19, 23
degenerative joint disease, 61
deli slices, 106, 111, 208-9, 211, 215
deli slices, soy, 211, 215

depression, 16, 45, 76, 94, 130, 153, 181, 182
desensitization, 59
designer diets, 24
Dexatrim, 26
dextrose, 117
DHA, 143
diabetes, 14, 15, 18, 19, 31, 65, **73**, 117
    correct diet for, 73
    low blood sugar and, 74
diarrhea, 25, 94, 96, 197
diet
    "foods", 24
    industry, 3
Diet Centers, 21, 23, 31
dieters, % who regain weight, 4
dieting
    as national obsession, 4
    defined, 29, 47
    fact review, 30
    facts about, 100
    lean body mass and, 101
    makes you fatter, 101
    metabolic rate and, 100
    money spent on, 4
    muscle loss due to, 9
    shakes and powders, 101
    statistics for, 22
    yo-yo, 4, 19, 31
digestion, **127**, 153
digestive enzymes, 128
    supplementation with, 151
digestive organs, **128**
digestive tract problems, 197
dinner, 209
dizziness, 26, 59, 88, 96
docosahexaenoic acid, 143
doctor
    things to say to, 54
    warning signs in, 55
    when to see, 198
doctors' role, 2, 3
dong quai, 80
drugs, 38, 50, 185
    causing weight gain, 13
    for dieting, 20, 26
    pregnancy and, 90
    with BioSlim, 26
duodenum, 96

eating
    a way to, 165
    when to begin, 122
    when to stop, 122
echinacea, and infections, 87
EFA, *See* Essential Fatty Acids
egg whites, 106, 111, 211, 215
eggplant, 61, 71, 105, 210
eggs, 42, 72, 106, 130, 197, 208-12, 215
eicosapentaenoic acid, 133, 143
electrocardiogram, 8
electrolipography, 8
electronic media, 2
emotions, weight gain and, 16
endive, 105, 210
endocrinologists & thyroid, 95
energy, 6, 32, 33
energy level
    not high enough, 195
    too high, 196
environmental sensitivities, 76
    fatigue from, 76
enzymes, 127, 130
EPA, 133, 143
ephedra, 143
    asthma and, 88
    dangers of, 144
essential amino acids, 130

Essential Fatty Acids, 7, 62, 69, 71, 78, 80, 83, 96, 133, **143**, 147, 150, 200
essential hypertension, 85
estrogen replacement, 89
exercise, 17

false hunger, 166
fat, 184
    added, 14
    gene, 17
    monounsaturated, 15
    number of calories in, 14
    slows down digestion, 15
    storage, 12, 13
    where it lies, 9
    why is there?, 6
fat cells, 12
fat-free deli slices, 106
fatigue, 25, 56, 59, 61, 94, 181, 203
    psychological disorders, 75
fatigue, chronic, 75
fats, 42, 107, **132**
    added, 15, 42, 69, 103, 107, 186, 207
    calculating intake, 134
    cancer and, 64
    effect on metabolic rate, 16
    heated, 134
    hydrogenated, 134
    saturated, 133
    trans fatty acids, 134
    unsaturated, 133
fat-soluble vitamins, 133
fear of success, 16
Federal Trade Commission, 21, 24, 31
fever, 35

feverfew, headaches and, 80
fiber, 69, 72, 84, 197
    heart disease and, 83
finasteride, 91
fish, 42, 72, 106, **113**, 130, 197, 208-9, 212
flour, 6, 14, 207, 212
    white, 41
fluids
    kidney stones and, 86
folic acid, 60, 64, 69, 71, 83, 90, **138**, 200
food
    allergies, 183
    allergies, in asthma, 87
    deep fried, avoiding, 123
    preparation, 120
    rating guide, 110
    timing, 121, 193
    to avoid, 116
Food Plan, 6, **102-103**, 189, 195
food sensitivities
    colitis and, 70
    headaches and, 80
food/diet imbalance, 181, 184
fowl, 130, 185
free radicals, 57
free T4, 95
french fries, 41
fructose, 6, 14, 131
fruit, 85, **115**
    juices, 116, 185, 208, 212
FTC, *See* Federal Trade Commission

galactosemia, 65
gallbladder, 31
gallbladder inflammation, 18
gallstones, 18, 23, **78**

and cholesterol, 78
gamma linolenic acid, 133
garlic, 69, 83, 85, 98, 105
gas, intestinal, 33, 197
gastritis, 96
gastroenteritis, 70
gastrointestinal disease, 31
ginkgo bilboa, 83
GLA, 62, 65, 133, 143
glucose, 131
    intolerance, 25
gluten, 70
glycogen, 127, 132
gout, 18, 86
government, 20
grains, 6, 14, 85
grapefruit, 24, 211
grapefruit seed extract, 98
growth hormone, **13**, 17, 19
    and aging, 13
gumbo soup, 210

habits, positive, 158
hay fever, 78
HDL, 67
headaches, **79**, 130, 181, 203
    constipation and, 80
    migraine, 79
    sinus, 79
health care, in America, 5
Health Management Resources, 21
heart, 23, 85
    attack, 81
    diabetes and, 73
    palpitations, 26
heart disease, 14, 18, 31, 77, **81**, 117, 130
    nutritional factors, 82
    prevention, 82

heartburn, 96
heavy metal toxicity, fatigue from, 75
Helicobacter, ulcers and, 96
hemorrhoidal veins, 83
hemorrhoids, 83
HEPA air filters, 88
herbal tea, 209
Herbamare, 212
hernias, 18
high blood pressure, 84
    biofeedback and, 85
hips, fat on 10
HIV, 203
hormonal dysfunction, 75
hormone replacement, 56, 89, 202
Horsetail, for silicon, 142
hot-dogs, soy & regular, 210
hunger
    false, 166
    scale, 169
    true, 167
hydrogenated fats, 134
hyperinsulinemia, 6, 13
hyperlipidemia, 25
hypersomnia, 94
hypertension. *See* high blood pressure
    essential, 85
hyperthyroidism, 93
hypnotherapy, 125
hypoglycemia, 79, 181
hypoparathyroidism, 65
hypotension, 25
hypothyroidism, 59, **93**, 94, 95, 96
    cholesterol levels and, 67

IBS. *See* irritable bowel syndrome
ice cream, 41, 117
ideal weight, 7
Imitrex, 79
immune system, 61, 203
indulging, 124
infectious disease, 75
IBD. *See* inflammatory bowel disease
inflammatory bowel disease, 70
inositol, 138
insomnia, 26, 36, 59, 94, 130
insulin, 6, 13, 14, 15, 42, 73, 107, 181
insulin resistance, 14, 73
intestinal gas, 197
intestines, 128
intimacy, avoiding, 45
invert sugar, 131
iodine, 83, 96, **142**
Ionamin, 26
iron, 59, 60, 71, 77, 90, **142**, 200, 201
   testing for, 60
iron deficiency, 59
irritable bowel syndrome, 70

Jenny Craig, 21, 23, 31
juices, fruit, 6, 107, 115, 185, 208, 212
junk food, 40, 118

kale, 211
ketosis, 25
kidney, 31, 61
kidney beans, 112
kidneys, 56, 73, 85
   stones, 85

lactobacillus, 71, 72, 78, 97, 98, 113, 150, 198, 204
lactose intolerance, 70, 113
lard, 117
laxatives, 72
LDL, 67
lean body weight, 8, 10
lecithin, 89
lemon juice, 113, 212
lens, of the eye, 65
lentil, 209, 211
lettuce, 105, 211
lightheadedness, 181
lima beans, 112
linoleic acid, 133
liposuction, 20, 27
liquid protein diet, 10
liver, 64, 118
   disease, 18
longevity, 153
loratadine, 13
lunch, 208
lung disease, 18
lung disorders, 86
lupus, 77
Lyme disease, 75

macadamia nuts, 15
magnesium, 59, 65, 69, 71, 77, 80, 83, 84, 86, 88, 89, 90, 93, **141**, 147, 150, 200
magnesium-potassium aspartate, 78
ma-huang, 143
maltose, 117
manganese, 69, 90, **142**
margarine, 41, 116, 207

mayonnaise, 41, 117, 207
McDonald's, 212
meal replacements, 20, 24, 26, 31, 101
meal size, cravings and, 187
meal timing, 108
meat, 42, 72, 87, 106, 111, **114**, 118, 124, 130, 185, 197, 208 red, 118
meat, protein, vs. spirulina, 121
medical profession, 2
    responsibilities of, 3
medications, weight gain &, 13
medicine, preventive, 3
Medifast, 21, 31
menopause, 79, 202
menstruation, 23
    changes, 202
    irregularities of, 18
menstruation, changes due to thyroid, 94
mental tools, 175
Meridia, 26
metabolic rate, 10, 12, 16, 30, **128**, 152
    advancing age and, 129
    age and, 129
    dieting and, 100
    in children, 39
    reduction of, 12
    thyroid and, 129
metabolism, 44, **128**
    basal, 13
    resting, 13
Micro Diet, 22, 23
micro-crystalline hydroxyapatite, 90
migraines, 79
milk, 37, 42, 72, 77, 80, 87, 97, 112, 118, 130, 196-7, 208-9, 211
    and colitis, 70
milk of magnesia, 72
milk, and childhood infections, 37
millet, 115
minerals, **141**
mirror, 9
mirror criteria, 8
mites, and asthma, 88
mitral valve prolapse, 83
molybdenum, **142**
mood, improvement in, 33
motivation, mastering, 162, 194
multiple sclerosis (MS), 75, 88
muscle(s), 8
    mass, 10, 30
    tension, 153
    weakness in, 88
mushrooms, 105
mustard, 212

n-acetyl-cysteine, 87
nails, brittle, 59
naturally thin, 165, 175
nausea, 56
niacin, 60, 69, 80, 83, **138**, 148
nightshades, 61, 71
nitrites, 87
nodules, 61
nut (or seed) butters
    how to use, 116
Nutri/System, 21, 23, 31
nutrition, 3, **126**
    deficiencies, 181, 183
    education on, 38
    in children, 39
    reversal of deficiencies, 33
nutritional supplements, 145
    additional, 150

effects of, 148
interactions among, 150
purpose of, 145
nuts, 71
nuts and seeds, **116**
Nystatin, 204

oat, 71
oatmeal, 14, 209
obesity, 7, 15
   as cause of fatigue, 76
   childhood, 39
   consequences of, 18
   Cushing's syndrome &, 56
   defined, 7
   gallstones and, 78
   in doctor, 55
   inevitability of, 39
   "normal" with age, 40
   overeating and, 127
obstructive pulmonary disease, 86
oil, 41, 116, 207
olive, and olive oil, 15
omega-3 fatty acids, 133, 143
omega-6 fatty acids, 133, 143
Optifast, 21, 31
osteoarthritis, 18, 61
osteoporosis, 89
   estrogen and, 89
   prevalence, 89
   smoking and, 90
   thyroid treatment and, 89
oxalate, 86
ozone depletion, 50

PABA, 138
pallor, 59
palpitations, 26
pancreas, 73, 128
pantothenic acid, 59, 60, 77, 88, **138**
pasta, 6, 14
peanut butter, 116-117
pears, 209
peas, 112, 211
peppermint, 113
peppers, 61, 71, 105
phentermine, 26
phenylalanine, 130
phenylpropanolamine, 26
phosphorus, 141
Physicians Weight Loss Centers, 21, 23
pituitary, 13, 95
PMS, 65, 79, 130
pneumonia, 35, 86
pollen, 37
pollution, 50
potassium, 85, 141
potato, 14, 61, 71, 107, 207-8, 212
potato chips, 41, 117
potatoes, 6
poultry, 42, 106, 111, **114**
Pounds Off diet bars, 20, 22
powders, 10, 20, 22, 24
pregnancy, 90, 201
   BioSlim and, 91
preventive medicine, 3
problems, solving, 191
processed food, 50
prostate, 64, **91**
   enlargement of, 91
protein, 14, 42, 86, 90, 106, **130**, 208
protein-carbohydrate balance, 6, 42, 106, 186, 208
psyllium, 72, 78, 84

puddings, 118
pulmonary hypertension, 26
pumpkin, 210
pyridoxal-5'-phosphate, 138
pyridoxine, 138

quercetin, 62, 65, 143
quinoa, 115

radiation, 50, 63
radishes, 105, 211
raisins, 211-2
RDA, 135
recognizable food, 104, 106
reflux, 97
relaxation therapy, 92
respiration, cellular, 59
restaurants, eating in, 122
retina, 65
rheumatoid arthritis, 61, 65, 77
rhubarb, 86
riboflavin, **137**
rice, 14, 24, 115, 197, 207, 212
    brown, 14
rye, 71

saccharose, 117, 131
SAD. *See* seasonal affective disorder
salad dressing, 41, 117, 123
salad, blended, 208
salt, 119, 184, 212
    headaches and, 79
saturated fats, 69
sausage, 208
saw palmetto, 91
scale, hunger, 169
sciatica, 18
seafood, 113

seasonal affective disorder, 16
seaweeds, 106, 111
secondary gain, 44
seizures, 130
selenium, 58, 64, 66, 69, 71, 83, 88, 140, **142**
self-destructive impulse, 45
seronoa repens, 91
sex drive, thyroid and, 94
sex hormone, 56
shakes, 10, 20, 24, 31, 101
shakes, diet, 22
sibutramine, 26
side benefits, of BioSlim, 34, 50, 149
silicon, 142
skin
    dry, 59
    fold thickness, 8
    sun exposure and, 92
    wrinkling, 92
sleep disorders, 19
SlimTone Formula, 145, **146**, 192, 195, 196, 201
    how to use, 146
    in pregnancy, 201
    after goals reached, 147
smoking, 46, 68, 70, 89
    and aging, 58
    and asthma, 88
    and lung disease, 87
    and osteoporosis, 90
    and pregnancy, 90
    and ulcer disease, 97
SOD (SuperOxide Dismutase), 62, 143
sodium, 85
soft drinks, 14, 41, 118, 208, 212
sore throat, 35

soups, 112
soy, 42, 106, 111, 208, 210, 211, 215
    milk, 118, 209, 211, 212
soybeans, 112
spinach, 86, 106, 209. 211
spirulina, 41, 42, 106, **121**, 130, 150, 208-9, 211, 215
spirulina, protein, vs. meat, 121
sprouts, 211
squash, 211
staphylococcus, 37
starvation, 6
steroids, 13, 35, 65
Stinging Nettle, & allergies, 59
stomach, 15, 64, 128
    stapling, 27
streptococcus, 37
stress, 16, **92**
    adrenals and, 56
    biofeedback and, 92
    ulcer disease and, 97
stroke, 81
sucrose, 14, 117, 131
sugar, 6, 14, 41, 69, 77, 80, 98, 105, 107, **117**, 131, 184, 186, 197, 212
    osteoporosis and, 90
    yeast and, 98
sugar
    refined, 71
    rush, 131
sulfur, 141
sumatryptan, 79
sunlight, depression and, 16
Super BioSlim, 5, 32, 109, 194, 195, **213**
superoxide dismutase, 143
Suprax, 36

surgery,
    for cancer, 63
    for obesity, 20, 27
Synthroid, 95
syphilis, 75

T7 (thyroid test), 95
tachycardia, 83
Taco Bell, 212
tahini, 116
tang kwei, 80
taurine, 85, 130
tea, herbal, 113, 209
television, and obesity, 39
therapeutic exercises, for back pain, 63
thermogenesis, food induced, 15, 16
thiamine, 137
thighs, fat on 10
thin, naturally, 175
thirst, 174
Thorazine, 65
thyroid, **93**, 181, 182, 199
    hormone deficiency, 93
    hormone excess, 93
    inflammation of, 94
    metabolic rate and, 129
    tests for, 94
    therapeutic trial for, 95
    women and, 199
thyroiditis, 77, 93, 94
TIA. *See* transient ischemic attacks
TMJ syndrome, 79
tobacco, 61
tofu, 114, 210
tomato, 61, 71, 106, 208-12
tools, mental, 175

tooth brushing, cravings and, 187
toxemia of pregnancy, 18
tranquilizers, 36
trans fatty acids, 83, 104, 134
    and heart disease, 83
transient ischemic attacks, 81
tricyclic antidepressants, 13
triglycerides, 6, 13, 18, 107
true hunger, 167
tryptophan, 130
    and the FDA, 130
TSH, 94, 95
tuberculosis, 37
turkey, 106, 111, 208-9, 211-2
turnip greens, 106

ulcers, 59, **96**
Ultra/Slim Fast, 22
    loathsome advertising, 23
Ultrafast, 21, 31
United Weight Control Corporation, 21
unsaturated fats, 67
unsaturated oils, & MS, 89
upper respiratory infection
    causes of, 38
uric acid, 25, 86
urine yellowing, 147, 149
uterine cancer
    and estrogen, 90

vaginitis, 98
vegetables, 14, 41, 85, 89, 105, **111**
    weight losing, 105
vicious circle, ending, 179
vinegar, 208, 212
vinegar, apple cider, 62

visual disturbances, 88
Vita/Min Plus, 145, **147**, 149, 192, 195, 196, 201
    importance of taking with food, 148
    in pregnancy, 201
    use of, 147
vitamin A, 59, 64, 71, 78, 83, 86, 87, 88, 97, **136**
vitamin B1, 60, **137**
vitamin B12, 60, 71, 77, 88, 89, 121, **137**, 138
vitamin B2, 60, 66, 86, **137**, 147
vitamin B3, **138**
vitamin B5, **138**
vitamin B6, 60, 62, 65, 69, 77, 80, 83, 84, 86, 88, 97, **138**, 200
vitamin C, 58, 59, 60, 62, 64, 66, 69, 71, 77, 78, 83, 84, 86, 87, 90, 93, 97, **138**, 140, 147, 151
vitamin D, 90, **139**
vitamin E, 58, 59, 60, 64, 66, 69, 78, 83, 84, 89, 97, **140**, 147, 151
vitamin K, **140**
vitamin U, 97
vitamins, **135**
    from diet, 135
vomiting, 96

water, 71, 113, **119**, 208, 215
    cravings and, 186
    constipation and, 72
    losses, in dieting, 22
water chestnuts, 106
watercress, 106
watermelon, 24
weakness, 56, 59, 181

weight loss
    too rapid, 195
    too slow, 191
weight loss, as health issue, 4
weight reaction categories, 44
Weight Watchers, 21, 23, 31
Western diet, 39, 40, 48
wheat, 71
    whole, 14, 114, 115, 207
wheezing, 87
white blood cells, 61
white flour, 41, 115, 117, 182, 207
white willow bark, 143
whole grains, 115, 207
Wilson's disease, 65

women
    special considerations, 199
    nutritional needs, 199
    thyroid function and, 199

yeast, 71
yeast infections, 203
yeast syndromes, 203
yogurt, 112, 113, 209, 211
yo-yo phenomenon, 110, 213

zinc, 66, 69, 71, 77, 80, 83, 87, 89, 91, 97, **142**
zucchini, 211